Good Housekeeping

Calorie Counter

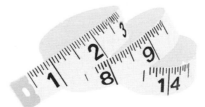

Contents

4 How to use this book
6 Calorie counting made easy
8 A healthy diet
14 How to read food labels
16 Calculating your BMI
18 How to offset your calories

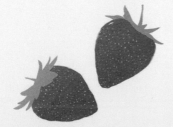

Calorie Counts

22 Bacon, ham & pork
24 Beans, lentils, nuts & seeds
26 Beef & beef dishes
28 Beverages
32 Biscuits (savoury) & cereal bars
34 Biscuits (sweet) & bars
36 Bread & bakery
38 Breakfast cereals
42 Cakes, pastries & buns
44 Cheese
46 Confectionery
50 Crisps & snacks
54 Eating out
60 Eggs
62 Fats & oils
64 Fish
66 Fish & seafood
68 Fish products & dishes
70 Fruit
76 Ice cream

80 Lamb
82 Milk
84 Offal
86 Pasta & pasta dishes
90 Pastry & savoury pies
92 Pizza
94 Poultry & game
98 Puddings
100 Rice, noodles & rice dishes
102 Salads
106 Sauces & dressings
108 Soft drinks
116 Soups
118 Spreads
120 Storecupboard ingredients
122 Takeaways
124 Vegetables
128 Vegetarian products
132 Yoghurt
132 Cream

134 My calorie counting chart
139 Body Mass Index (BMI) chart
140 Calorie swaps
142 Useful websites

How to use this book

Whether you want to lose weight, maintain your weight or gain weight, this book will help you get more calorie savvy. It lists the calorie values of more than 1,200 popular foods and drinks, including staples, such as milk, bread and meat, as well as many branded products, takeaways and restaurant dishes.

Calorie counting may sound old hat, but any nutritionist will tell you that when it comes to weight control, calories always count. Take in more calories than your body uses and you will gain weight as the body stores fat; use more calories than you take in and the weight comes off. This is the principle behind all diets, whether they are low fat, low carb or any other combination of nutrients. To lose weight, you have to consume fewer calories than you burn!

This book is about more than calories. It also gives you the amounts of fat, saturated fat, carbohydrate, protein and fibre per portion for each food. With this information you will see which nutrients each food contributes to your daily intake and so it will help you to plan a healthy diet. You will be able to tally your daily calorie and nutritional intake. Keep a note of what you eat and drink, and then look up each item in the calorie charts and add the figures together. To lose weight, you should try to keep within your daily calorie allowance (page 7); to gain weight you should aim to eat more than your daily calorie expenditure (page 7).

You can also use this book to help you plan your day's food, your weekly shopping and even your meals when eating out. Knowing the calorific value of foods in advance allows you to choose lower calorie and healthier options. Use it to compare similar types of foods or find out how many calories may be hidden in your favourite meals.

The foods are grouped into categories – fruit, vegetables, bread and bakery, pasta, confectionery, soft drinks, eating out and so on – to make it as easy as possible to locate a particular item.

The foods in each category are listed alphabetically so that you can find them easily.

The values for unbranded foods have been obtained from McCance & Widdowson's *The Composition of Foods* (6th summary edition and subsequent supplements), and have been reproduced under the terms of the Open Government Licence. Those for branded items have been obtained from the websites of supermarkets and food manufacturers.

Calories and nutrients are given per standard portion to make life as easy as possible! It means that you don't have to weigh your food or calculate anything. But if you need to know the calories in a different-sized portion,

multiply the calories given in this book by the weight of your portion, then divide by the weight given for the standard portion.

It has not been possible to include every food and every brand, but we have tried to give a representative sample of generic foods and brands under each category. If you cannot find a particular item here, you may be able to use the values for a similar product. The nutritional values are up to date at the time of publication but it should be noted that values may change from time to time, because manufacturers frequently change their formulations and amend recipes. Similarly, new products frequently appear on the supermarket shelves and existing ones are withdrawn.

Calorie counting made easy

Counting calories is the easiest way to control your diet and lose weight. It's scientifically proven, it gives you maximum flexibility and is guaranteed to help you shed pounds – provided you stick to your daily calorie allowance!

Losing weight isn't rocket science. By taking in fewer calories from food and drink than you burn through your daily activity, you will drop pounds. And that's where this book can really help. It gives you up-to-date calorie and nutritional information for hundreds of branded and unbranded foods in different categories, to make calorie counting as easy as possible. You are then free to eat anything as long as it is within your daily calorie allowance.

Start subtracting. To lose 0.5kg (1lb) a week, you need to create a calorie deficit of just 500 calories a day. This isn't as daunting as it seems. You can achieve this by foregoing a couple of chocolate biscuits and a glass of wine to save 300 calories; and walking for 40 minutes to burn another 200 calories. Losing 0.5kg (1lb) a week amounts to 7kg (1 stone) in 14 weeks, or 26kg (4 stone) in a year.

It's calories that count. Many diets restrict your intake of one particular nutrient, usually carbohydrates or fat. But the results of a 2012 study published in the *American Journal of Clinical Nutrition* suggest that when it comes to weight loss, it's simply calories that count (although, of course, eating a good balance of nutrients is important). Provided they stuck to their daily calorie allowance, dieters lost the same amount of weight in six months whether they cut carbs or fat, or upped protein. The key, it seems, is to find a plan that you can comfortably live with, rather than attempting to lose weight periodically with strict diets that are hard to maintain.

What is a calorie? Everyone talks about calories as if they are something contained in food. In fact, a calorie is a measure of energy, just as a kilo is a measure of weight and a mile is a measure of distance. In scientific terms, one calorie is the amount of energy (heat) required to increase the temperature of 1g of water by 1°C.

Calories, kilocalories, kilojoules – what's the difference? All of these terms crop up on food labels, which can be a bit confusing! Suffice to say that the scientifically defined calorie is a very small energy unit that is inconvenient to use because an average serving of any food typically provides thousands of these calories. For this reason, when speaking about food in the everyday sense, we say 'calorie' when we mean 'kilocalorie'; for example, a food label may declare a portion of food contains 100kcal but we would probably say 100 calories. You'll also see food energy measured in joules or kilojoules on food labels, which is the SI (International Unit System) unit for energy. 1 kcal is equivalent to 4.2kJ.

Here's how you can reduce your calorie intake to kick-start weight loss:

1. Find your daily calorie expenditure

Your calorie needs depend on your genetic make-up, age, weight, body composition, and your daily activity. They will differ from one day to the next and as you grow older. As a rough guide, it's around 2,000 calories a day for an average woman and 2,500 for a man. For a more accurate estimate of the number of calories you use during daily living and exercise, go to http://nutritiondata.self.com/tools/calories-burned and enter your gender, age, weight, height, lifestyle and details of daily exercise.

2. Work out your daily calorie allowance

Trim 500 calories off that total. For example, if your daily calorie burn is 2,000, then subtract 500 to get 1,500 calories. This is your daily calorie allowance, which will produce a weight loss of 0.5–1kg (1–2lb) per week. Don't try to lose more than this, otherwise you risk fatigue, excessive muscle loss and a significant drop in your metabolic rate, making weight loss harder. Record what you eat and tally your calorie intake with the help of this book. You will find some blank calorie counting charts at the end of the book.

A healthy diet

Counting calories is important when you're trying to drop pounds, but you also need to make sure your diet is healthy and contains a good balance of nutrients. Here's what you need to eat each day.

Fat

Your body needs fat from foods to provide fuel and help to keep cell membranes healthy. It is also a source of vitamins A, D and E, and essential fatty acids (omega-3s and omega-6s), which the body cannot make itself.

However, eating too much fat can be unhealthy because – compared to carbohydrate and protein – it is very high in calories. It is therefore important for your health that you watch the amount of fatty foods you eat. Aim to replace some of the unhealthy saturated fat in your diet with healthier unsaturated fat, as this will provide a better balance and will be beneficial for your heart.

There are three main types of fat – saturated, monounsaturated and polyunsaturated – and most foods contain a combination of these three. Foods also contain other fats, as described right:

Saturated fat can raise blood cholesterol levels, which increases the chance of developing heart disease. It is found in fatty meat, sausages, burgers, bacon, butter, chocolate, cheese, palm oil ('vegetable fat'), and foods made from butter or vegetable fat (such as pies, biscuits and cakes).

Trans fats are found in *hydrogenated fat*, formed when hydrogen is added to liquid oils to make them solid. They increase blood levels of LDL cholesterol ('bad' cholesterol), harden your arteries and increase your risk of heart disease. Many manufacturers have removed these fats, but high levels may still be found in deep-fried fast foods, cakes, biscuits and doughnuts. Check the label for hydrogenated fat.

Monounsaturates and poly-unsaturates are both types of unsaturated fat. These don't raise blood cholesterol in the same way as saturated fats and they provide you with the essential fatty acids that the body needs.

Monounsaturated fats are found in olive oil, margarine made with olive oil, avocados, nuts, seeds, peanut butter and rapeseed oil.

Polyunsaturated fats are found in sunflower oil, corn oil, safflower oil, margarine made with sunflower oil, nuts and seeds.

Omega-3 fatty acids are essential for regulating blood pressure and blood clotting and for boosting immunity. They help to reduce the risk of heart disease and are found in oily fish, walnuts, pumpkin seeds, flaxseed oil, rapeseed oil and omega-3 eggs.

Omega-6 fatty acids are important for healthy skin and hormones. They are found in most vegetable oils, vegetable oil margarine, and products made from them. Use sparingly, as a high intake will block the uptake of omega-3 fats.

Protein

We need to eat protein to make and repair body cells, as well as to manufacture enzymes, hormones and antibodies. The richest sources include meat, fish, poultry, eggs, milk, cheese and yogurt, and good levels are also found in beans, lentils, nuts, seeds, Quorn, tofu and cereals. When two or more plant proteins are combined (such as beans on toast) the overall protein value increases.

Carbohydrate

Sugars and starch provide energy for daily activities as well as fuel for exercise. Your brain, nervous system and heart need a constant supply of carbohydrate in order to function properly. Generally, carbohydrates in fibre-rich unprocessed foods, such as wholegrains, potatoes, beans, lentils, fruit and vegetables, provide longer-lasting energy and help you feel full for longer. These foods should make up most of your carbohydrate intake.

Fibre

The digestive system requires fibre from foods for it to work properly, and fibre is also useful for weight control. There are two kinds: insoluble and soluble. Most plant foods contain both, but proportions vary. Good sources of insoluble fibre include whole grains (such as brown rice, wholemeal bread) and vegetables. These foods help speed the passage of food through your gut, preventing constipation and bowel problems, and they make you feel full after eating. Soluble fibre – found in oats, beans, lentils, fruit and vegetables – reduces harmful LDL cholesterol levels, and it helps to control blood glucose levels by slowing glucose absorption. It also reduces hunger and improves appetite control. A healthy diet should contain at least 18g (¾oz) a day.

Salt and sodium

On a food label, salt is often listed as sodium, and 1g of sodium is roughly the same as 2.5g of salt. It's the sodium that can lead to health problems such as high blood pressure, increasing your risk of stroke and coronary heart disease. Adults should not have more than 6g (about 1 tsp) of salt per day.

The eatwell plate

To help you eat healthily, the government has devised an eating system called the eatwell plate, based on the five food groups:
- Bread, rice, potatoes, pasta and other starchy foods
- Fruit and vegetables
- Milk and dairy foods
- Meat, fish, eggs, beans and other non-dairy sources of protein
- Foods and drinks high in fat and/or sugar

The eatwell plate shows the different types of food you need to eat – and in what proportions – to have a well balanced and healthy diet. You should try to eat a wide variety of foods from the first four groups every day, and limit the amount you eat from the fifth group.

It's a good idea to try to get this balance right every day, but you don't need to do it at every meal. And you might find it easier to get the balance right over a longer period, say a week. Based on the eatwell plate, you should try to eat:

Bread, rice, potatoes, pasta and other starchy foods

Eat these foods at each meal

These foods should make up roughly a third of the food you eat. Try to choose wholegrain varieties where you can, such as wholemeal bread and pasta, wholegrain breakfast cereals and wholegrain rice. A portion is:
- 2 slices of bread
- 5 tablespoons (180g) pasta or rice
- 40g bowl of breakfast cereal
- 1 fist-sized (150g) potato

Fruit and vegetables

Eat at least 5 portions a day

These foods should make up about a third of the food you eat each day. Aim to eat a variety of fruit and vegetables each day. Fresh, frozen, tinned, dried and juiced all count.

A portion is 80g or any of these:

- 1 apple, banana, pear or orange
- 2 small fruits e.g. satsumas, plums, apricots
- 3 heaped tablespoons of vegetables
- a dessert bowl of salad
- a glass (150ml) of fruit juice (counts as a maximum of one portion a day)

Milk and dairy foods

Eat 2 or 3 portions a day

Foods in this group include milk, cheese and yoghurt. Choose lower-fat options where available, such as skimmed milk. Or you could have just a small amount of the high-fat varieties less often.

A portion is:

- 200ml milk
- A small pot of yoghurt
- A matchbox sized (40g) piece of cheese

Meat, fish, eggs, beans and other non-dairy sources of protein

Eat 2 portions a day

Try to eat some foods from this group each day and aim for at least two portions of fish a week, including a portion of oily fish. Some types of meat can be high in saturated fat so try to choose leaner cuts where possible and trim excess fat. Beans, peas and lentils are good alternatives to meat because they're naturally low in fat, and they're high in fibre, protein, and vitamins and minerals.

A portion is:

- A piece of meat, chicken or fish the size of a deck of cards (70g)
- 2 eggs
- 2 heaped tablespoons of beans or lentils
- 2 tablespoons (25g) nuts or seeds

Foods and drinks high in fat and/or sugar

Eat only small amounts of these foods

These foods include cakes, biscuits, spreads, crisps, sugar, confectionery and soft drinks. Cutting down on these types of food could help you control your weight because they contain lots of calories.

Vitamins and minerals

Vitamins support the immune system, help the brain function and convert food into energy. They are important for healthy skin and hair, controlling growth and balancing hormones. Some vitamins – the B vitamins and vitamin C – must be provided by the diet daily, as they cannot be stored.

Minerals are needed for structural and regulatory functions, including bone strength, haemoglobin manufacture, fluid balance and muscle contraction.

Mineral	Use	Best food sources
Calcium	Builds bone and teeth. For blood clotting, nerve and muscle function	Milk and dairy products; sardines; dark green leafy vegetables; pulses; Brazil nuts; almonds; figs; sesame seeds
Iron	For the formation of red blood cells and for oxygen transport. Prevents anaemia	Meat and offal; wholegrain cereals; fortified breakfast cereals; pulses; green leafy vegetables; nuts; sesame and pumpkin seeds
Zinc	For a healthy immune system, wound healing, and skin and cell growth	Eggs; wholegrain cereals; meat; nuts and seeds
Magnesium	For healthy bones, muscle and nerve function and for cell formation	Cereals; fruit; vegetables; milk; nuts and seeds
Potassium	For fluid balance, and for muscle and nerve function	Fruit; vegetables; cereals; nuts and seeds
Sodium	For fluid balance, and for muscle and nerve function	Salt; processed meat; ready meals; sauces; soup; cheese; bread
Selenium	An antioxidant that helps protect against heart disease and cancer	Cereals; vegetables; dairy products

Vitamin	Use	Best food sources
A	For vision in dim light; healthy skin and linings of the digestive tract, nose and throat	Full-fat dairy products; meat; offal; oily fish; margarine
Beta-carotene	An antioxidant that protects against certain cancers; converts into vitamin A	Fruit and vegetables e.g. apricots, peppers, tomatoes, mangoes, broccoli, squash, carrots, watercress
Vitamin B_1 (thiamin)	Releases energy from carbohydrates. For healthy nerves and digestive system	Wholemeal bread and cereals; pulses; meat; sunflower seeds
Vitamin B_2 (riboflavin)	Releases energy from carbohydrates. For healthy skin, eyes and nerves.	Milk and dairy products; meat; eggs, soya products
Vitamin B_3 (niacin)	Releases energy from carbohydrates; Healthy skin, nerves and digestion.	Meat and offal; nuts; milk and dairy products; eggs; wholegrain cereals
Vitamin B_6 (pyridoxine)	Metabolises protein, carbohydrate, fat. For red blood cell manufacture and a healthy immune system	Pulses; nuts; eggs; cereals; fish; bananas
Folic acid	Formation of DNA and red blood cells. Reduces risk of spina bifida in developing babies	Green leafy vegetables; yeast extract; pulses; nuts; citrus fruit
Vitamin B_{12}	Formation of red blood cells. For energy metabolism	Milk and dairy products; meat; fish; fortified breakfast cereals; soya products; yeast extract
Vitamin C	Healthy connective tissue, bones, teeth, blood vessels, gums and teeth. Promotes immune function. Helps iron absorption	Fruit and vegetables e.g. raspberries, blackcurrants, kiwi, oranges, peppers, broccoli, cabbage, tomatoes
Vitamin D	Builds strong bones. Needed to absorb calcium and phosphorus	Sunlight; oily fish; fortified margarine and breakfast cereals; eggs
Vitamin E	Antioxidant which helps protect against heart disease; promotes normal cell growth and development	Vegetable oils; oily fish; nuts; seeds; egg yolk; avocado

How to read food labels

Food labels provide useful information, but they can be confusing. Here's how to decipher them.

Read the list of ingredients

These are listed in descending order of weight; that is, the most to the least. If an ingredient is mentioned in the name of the product, such as the apple in 'apple pie', or is shown on the label, the amount of the ingredient in the food must be given as a percentage.

Read the nutrition label

The nutrients below must be listed per 100g or per 100ml:

- Energy (Kcals)
- Fat (g)
- Protein (g)
- Carbohydrate (g)

Food manufacturers can include more nutritional information, but if a food product makes a health claim for a specific nutrient, the relevant information must be listed; for example, if a food is described as low salt, the salt content must be given.

Read the Traffic Light or Guideline Daily Amount (GDA) labelling

Traffic light labels are the Food Standards Agency-approved labelling system, and they tell you whether the food has high, medium or low amounts of each of the listed nutrients in 100g of the food:

Green is used to show the food is low in that nutrient;
Amber signals that the product contains medium levels of that nutrient; and
Red represents high amounts and warns shoppers not to consume much.

Many of the foods with traffic light colours will have a mixture of red, amber and greens. The idea is, when you're choosing between similar products, to go for more greens and ambers, and fewer reds.

Guideline Daily Amounts (GDAs) are a guide to how much energy and key nutrients the average healthy person needs in order to have a balanced diet. The GDAs for the most important nutrients listed on food labels are: GDAs show how much of that nutrient is in a portion of food and are a guide and a maximum. If you are a normal weight you can aim to reach the GDA for calories, but try to eat no more than the GDAs for fat, saturates, salt and sugars.

	Men	**Women**
Fat (total)	95g	70g
of which saturates	30g	20g
Salt	6g	6g
Sugar*	120g	90g

* Total sugars includes sugars occurring naturally in foods as well as added sugars

Read the nutrition claims

It's important to understand these claims, because a chocolate rice breakfast cereal, for example, could claim to be low in fat, but it could also be high in sugar and calories.

A general rule is to treat these claims with caution. Something that claims to be lower in fat may still contain the same number of calories as other versions. It is best to decide whether a food is suitable by comparing the nutritional information of products.

'Low calorie'	Contains less than 40 calories per 100g
'Reduced calorie'	Contains at least 25% less than the standard version
'Low fat'	Contains less than 3g of fat per 100g (for food) or 1.5g of fat per 100ml (for liquids)
'Reduced fat'	Contains 25% less fat than a similar product.
'Less than 5% fat'	Contains less than 5g of fat per 100g of the food
'No added sugar'	No sugars have been added as an ingredient. But the product may still contain high levels of natural sugars from e.g. fruit juice or dried fruit
'Low sugar'	Contains no more than 5g sugar per 100g
'Reduced sugar'	Contains 25% less sugar than a similar product
'Lite' or 'light'	No legal definition

Calculating your BMI

Carrying too much weight increases your risk of high blood pressure, type-2 diabetes, heart disease and some types of cancer. To get a general picture of your health risk and determine a realistic weight goal, you can calculate your Body Mass Index (BMI) (see page 139).

What is my BMI?

Your BMI expresses your weight in relation to your height and works out whether you are overweight, underweight or just right for your height. People are classed as obese if they have a body mass index of over 30. They are overweight if it is 25–30. A BMI between 18.5 and 24.9 has the lowest health risk. To work out your BMI, divide your weight (kg) by the square of your height (m^2):

16

		Example
A	My weight = __ kg	71 kg
B	My height = __ m	1.65 m
C	My height^2 = (B) x (B) = __	1.65 x 1.65 = 2.72
D	MY BMI = A ÷ C = __	71 ÷ 2.72 = 26

Alternatively, you can calculate your BMI from the chart on page 139. First select your height then select your weight. Select the nearest value(s) to your own if they are not displayed on the chart. Your body mass index will be listed at the top of the BMI chart.

What it means

BMI less than 18.5: underweight. It's important to avoid being underweight as it can affect your ability to fight infection and recover from illness. It can also weaken your muscles – including your heart. If you're losing weight without trying, talk to your GP or practice nurse to make sure there aren't any other problems causing this

BMI 18.5–24.9: healthy weight. You are a healthy weight for your height. But you also check your waist measurement (see page 17). Aim to keep within a healthy weight range by eating a balanced diet and taking regular exercise.

BMI 25–29.9: overweight. Being overweight increases your risk of developing coronary heart disease, type

2 diabetes, certain cancers and high blood pressure. Keeping to a healthy weight will help you control your blood pressure and cholesterol levels. Aim to exercise more and eat fewer calories towards a healthier weight.

BMI more than 30: obese. As your BMI increases, your risk of developing coronary heart disease, type 2 diabetes and certain cancers increases. It is important that you take steps to reduce your weight. Aim to exercise more and eat fewer calories; read *Good Housekeeping Drop a Dress Size* for easy exercise ideas that you can build into your daily routine. As BMI is based on weight and height, by losing weight you will reduce your BMI and your risk of ill-health.

Waist management

The BMI is a useful method but it doesn't take into account where fat is stored in your body. This is important because 'apple' shaped people (with most of their fat stored around the abdomen) are more at risk of developing obesity-related diseases such as type-2 diabetes, high blood pressure and heart disease, than 'pear' shapes who have most of their fat on their hips. The BMI also does not allow for how much muscle you have. The following tests will help you find out your health risk:

1. Measure your waist:
This tells you roughly the amount of fat you carry in your abdomen and is regarded as more accurate than BMI in predicting type-2 diabetes risk. For women, if your waist measures more than 80cm (32in), or for men more than 94cm (37in), you need to lose weight.

2. Divide your waist measurement by your hip measurement:
This will tell you whether you are an apple or a pear shape. If the figure is greater than 0.85 for women or 0.95 for men, you are an apple shape and more at risk from diseases linked to obesity.

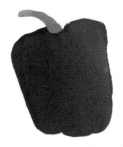

How to offset your calories

Being active is an important part of any weight-loss or weight-maintenance programme. When you're active, your body uses more energy (calories). And when you burn more calories than you consume, you lose weight.

Combining calorie counting with exercise means you will lose weight more easily and you will have so much more energy. *Good Housekeeping Drop a Dress Size* has lots of easy exercises and ideas to get you moving.

How much exercise? To lose weight, you should aim to be active for at least 60 minutes most days of the week, according to national guidelines. Anything that makes your heart beat faster counts: brisk walking, cycling, swimming or dancing. The key is to build a little more activity into your day.

Break up your activity. Fortunately, you don't have to do the whole lot at once to get benefits. Instead, you can build up the time over the course of

the day; for example, three 10-minute sessions of exercise produce the same results as one 30-minute session. Small changes can give big results. Look for small ways to add more activity to your day. Walking just one mile burns around 100 calories – equivalent to a chocolate biscuit, and this adds up to 36,500 calories or 10kg (22lb) of weight loss in a year.

Burn calories. Knowing the number of calories you burn in conjuction with a sensible diet can help you lose weight. This chart, which is based on a person weighing 59kg (9 stone 4lb) shows the number of calories burned during various activities. To lose 0.5kg (1lb), you must burn 3,500 more calories than you take in as food.

Six more reasons to get moving

There are many other great reasons for getting more active. Here are just some of them:

1. You'll feel less tired and have bags more energy.
2. Your body will be better able to fight off germs, which make you ill.
3. You'll feel better about yourself – and you'll look better too.
4. Your heart and lungs will become stronger.
5. Your muscles will become toned.
6. You'll cope better under stress.

Activity	Calories burned in 30 minutes
Aerobics (low impact)	149
Badminton	195
Cycling, 10mph (6 minutes/mile)	162
Dancing	130
Gardening	117
Hiking	202
Housework	117
Jogging, 6mph (10 minutes/mile)	299
Rowing machine	234
Running, 10mph 6 minutes/mile	455

Activity	Calories burned in 30 minutes
Shopping	78
Squash	266
Stair-climber machine	208
Step aerobics	189
Swimming (slow)	156
Swimming (fast)	292
Table Tennis	117
Tennis	208
Walking, 3mph (20 minutes/mile)	104
Weight training	247

12 EASY FOOD SWAPS
On page 140 We give you some easy ways to save calories by opting for lower-calorie alternatives.

Calorie Counts

Bacon, Ham & Pork	Av Portion	Calories	Fat, g
BACON			
Back rashers, grilled	15g (1 rasher)	43	3.0
Collar joint, boiled	85g	276	23
Gammon joint, trimmed, boiled	85g	142	5.0
Loin steak, grilled	100g	191	10
Streaky rashers, grilled	20g (1 rasher)	67	5.0
HAM			
Parma	45g	100	6.0
Premium	23g	30	1.0
PORK			
Belly joint, roasted	110g	322	24
Fillet slices, grilled	120g	214	6.0
Leg joint, roasted	90g	194	9.0
Leg joint, roasted, trimmed	90g	164	5.0
Loin chops, grilled	120g	308	19
Loin chops, grilled, trimmed	120g	221	8.0
Loin chops, roasted	75g	226	14
Loin joint, roasted	90g	228	15
Loin steaks, fried	20g	331	22
Mince	90g	172	9.0
Sausages, fried	45g (1 sausage)	139	11
Sausages, grilled	45g (1 sausage)	132	10
Spare rib joint, roasted	90g	234	16
Spare rib joint, roasted, trimmed	90g	181	8.0
Steaks, grilled	135g	267	10
Steaks, grilled, trimmed	135g	228	5.0

*No information available
Tr trace quantities<0.1g

Saturated fat, g	Carbohydrate, g	Protein, g	Fibre, g
1.2	0	3.5	0
9.0	0	17	0
1.8	0	25	0
3.5	0	26	0
2.0	0	4.8	0
1.9	0	12	0
0.4	0.1	4.9	0
8.1	0	28	0
2.3	0	40	0
3.2	0	28	0
1.7	0	30	0
6.7	0	35	0
2.6	0	38	0
5.3	0	24	0
5.3	0	27	0
7.2	0	33	0
3.5	0	22	0
3.8	4.5	6.3	0.3
3.6	4.4	6.5	0.3
6.0	0	22	0
2.9	0	27	0
3.6	0	44	0
1.8	0	46	0

Beans, lentils, nuts & seeds	Av Portion	Calories	Fat, g
BEANS & LENTILS			
Baked beans	200g (1 small can)	162	1.0
Baked beans, reduced sugar	200g (1 small can)	148	1.0
Black-eye beans, dried, boiled	120g (4 tbsp)	139	1.0
Broad beans, boiled	120g (4 tbsp)	58	1.0
Butter beans, canned, drained	120g (4 tbsp)	92	1.0
Chickpeas, canned, drained	120g (4 tbsp)	138	3.0
Lentils, green or brown, dried, boiled	120g (4 tbsp)	126	1.0
Lentils, red, dried, boiled	120g (4 tbsp)	120	0
Pinto beans, dried, boiled	120g (4 tbsp)	164	1.0
Red kidney beans	120g (4 tbsp)	120	1.0
NUTS & SEEDS			
Almonds	25g (a small handful)	153	14
Brazil nuts	25g (a small handful)	171	17
Cashew nuts	25g (a small handful)	143	12
Chestnuts	25g (a small handful)	43	1.0
Coconut, dessicated	25g (a small handful)	151	16
Hazelnuts	25g (a small handful)	163	16
Macadamia nuts	25g (a small handful)	187	19
Peanuts, roasted, salted	25g (a small handful)	151	13
Pecan nuts	25g (a small handful)	172	18
Pine nuts	25g (a small handful)	172	17
Pistachio nuts	25g (a small handful)	150	14
Pumpkin seeds	15g (1 tbsp)	85	7.0
Sesame seeds	15g (1 tbsp)	90	0
Sunflower seeds	15g (1 tbsp)	87	7.0
Walnuts	25g (a small handful)	172	17

*No information available
Tr trace quantities<0.1g

Saturated fat, g	Carbohydrate, g	Protein, g	Fibre, g
0.2	30	9.6	7.0
0.2	26	11	7.6
0.2	24	11	4.2
0.1	6.7	6.1	6.5
0.1	16	7.1	5.5
0.4	19	8.6	4.9
0.1	20	11	4.6
0	21	9.1	2.3
0.1	29	11	*
0.1	21	8.3	7.4
1.1	1.7	5.3	1.9
4.1	0.8	3.5	1.1
2.4	4.5	4.4	0.8
0.1	9.1	0.5	1.0
13	9.1	0.5	1.0
1.2	1.5	3.5	1.6
2.8	1.2	2.0	1.3
2.4	1.8	6.1	1.5
1.4	1.5	2.3	1.2
1.1	1.0	3.5	0.5
1.9	2.0	4.5	1.5
1.1	2.3	3.7	0.8
1.2	0.1	2.7	1.2
0.7	2.8	3.0	0.9
1.4	0.8	3.7	0.9

Beef & beef dishes	Av Portion	Calories	Fat, g
BEEF			
Beefburgers, fried	50g	165	12
Beefburgers, grilled	50g	163	12
Braising steak	140g	304	16
Fillet steak, fried	150g	288	13
Fillet steak, fried, trimmed	150g	276	12
Fillet steak, grilled	150g	300	14
Fillet steak, grilled, trimmed	150g	282	12
Mince	140g	286	20
Mince, lean	140g	244	13
Rump steak, grilled	150g	306	14
Sausages, fried	45g	126	9.0
Sausages, grilled	45g	125	9.0
Sirloin steak, fried, trimmed	175g	331	14
Sirloin steak, fried	175g	408	25
Sirloin steak, grilled	175g	373	22
Sirloin steak, grilled, trimmed	175g	308	13
Stewing steak, lean	140g	259	9.0
Topside, roasted	90g	200	10
Topside, roasted, trimmed	90g	158	5.0
BEEF DISHES			
Beef bourguignon	260g	317	16
Beef casserole	300g	408	20
Beef curry	350g	480	23
Chilli con carne	220g	211	9.0
Shepherd's pie	310g	347	18
Steak & kidney pie	160g	517	34

*No information available
Tr trace quantities<0.1g

Saturated fat, g	Carbohydrate, g	Protein, g	Fibre, g
5.3	0.1	14	0
5.4	0.1	13	0
6.7	0	41	0
5.9	0	42	0
5.1	0	42	0
6.6	0	43	0
5.4	0	44	0
8.7	0	27	0
5.9	0	31	0
7.8	0	44	0
3.4	5.6	6.1	0
3.6	5.9	6.0	0
6.0	0	50	0
11	0	47	0
9.8	0	43	0
6.0	0	47	0
3.2	0	45	0
4.3	0	27	0
1.9	0	29	0
5.4	6.5	36	1.0
8.2	14	45	*
11	22	47	4.2
4.2	16	17	3.1
6.8	29	19	2.2
13	41	15	1.4

Beverages	Av Portion	Calories	Fat, g
ALCOHOLIC DRINKS			
Bacardi Breezer	275ml, 1 bottle	96	0
Bailey's Original Irish Cream	25ml, 1 measure	82	3.3
Beer, bitter, draught	300ml, ½ pint	96	0
Brandy	25ml, 1 measure	56	0
Champagne	175ml, 1 glass	133	0
Cider, dry	300ml, ½ pint	108	0
Cider, sweet	300ml, ½ pint	126	0
Gin	25ml, 1 measure	56	0
Guinness	300ml, ½ pint	90	0
Lager	300ml, ½ pint	87	0
Liqueurs, high strength e.g. Drambuie, Pernod, Cointreau, Grand Marnier	25ml, 1 measure	79	0
Liqueurs, low–medium strength, e.g. Tia Maria, cherry brandy	25ml, 1 measure	66	0
Port	50ml, 1 glass	79	0
Red wine	175ml, 1 glass	119	0
Rose wine	175ml, 1 glass	124	0
Rum	25ml, 1 measure	56	0
Sherry, dry	50ml, 1 glass	58	0
Sherry, sweet	50ml, 1 glass	68	0
Vermouth, dry	50ml, 1 measure	55	0
Vermouth, sweet	50ml, 1 measure	76	0
Vodka	25ml, 1 measure	56	0
Whisky	25ml, 1 measure	56	0
White wine, dry	175ml, 1 glass	116	0
White wine, medium	175ml, 1 glass	130	0
White wine, sparkling	175ml, 1 glass	130	0
White wine, sweet	175ml, 1 glass	165	0

*No information available
Tr trace quantities<0.1g

Saturated fat, g	Carbohydrate, g	Protein, g	Fibre, g
0	8.3	0	0
*	6.3	0.8	0
0	6.9	0.9	0
0	0	0	0
0	2.4	0	0
0	7.8	0	0
0	13	0	0
0	0	0	0
0	4.5	1.2	0
0	4.5	0.6	0
0	6.1	0	0
0	8.2	0	0
0	6.0	0	0
0	0.4	0	0
0	4.4	0	0
0	0	0	0
0	0.7	0	0
0	3.5	0	0
0	1.5	0	0
0	7.9	0	0
0	0	0	0
0	0	0	0
0	1.1	0	0
0	5.3	0	0
0	8.9	0	0
0	10	0	0

Beverages	Av Portion	Calories	Fat, g
HOT DRINKS			
Filter Coffee, black	200ml	4	0
Filter coffee with semi-skimmed milk	200ml	14	0.3
Filter coffee with whole milk	200ml	16	0.8
Instant coffee, black	200ml	0	0
Instant coffee with semi-skimmed milk	200ml	14	0.3
Instant coffee with whole milk	200ml	16	0.8
Green tea	200ml	0	0
Herbal tea	200ml	2	0
Tea with semi-skimmed milk	200ml	14	0.3
Tea with whole milk	200ml	16	0.8
Hot chocolate with semi-skimmed milk	200ml	146	4.0
Hot chocolate with whole milk	200ml	180	8.0
Cocoa with semi-skimmed milk	200ml	114	4.0
Cocoa with whole milk	200ml	152	8.0
Latte with semi-skimmed milk	200ml	143	5.1
Latte with whole milk	200ml	172	8.4
Cappucino with semi-skimmed milk	200ml	97	3.4
Cappucino with whole milk	200ml	116	5.6
Mocha with semi-skimmed milk and whipped cream	200ml	273	13
Mocha with whole milk and whipped cream	200ml	297	16

*No information available
Tr trace quantities<0.1g

Saturated fat, g	Carbohydrate, g	Protein, g	Fibre, g
0	0.6	0.4	0
0.1	1.4	1.2	
0.2	1.4	1.2	0
0	0	0	0
0.1	1.4	1.2	0
0.2	1.4	1.2	0
0	0	0	0
0	0.4	0	0
0.1	1.4	1.2	0
0.2	1.4	1.2	0
2.5	1.4	1.0	0
5.2	21	7.0	0
2.4	14	7.0	0
5.2	14	6.8	0
2.6	15	9.5	0
4.8	15	9.1	0
1.7	10	6.4	0
3.2	10	6.1	0
7.7	33	9.8	0
9.5	33	9.5	0

Biscuits (savoury) & cereal bars	Av Portion	Calories	Fat, g
SAVOURY BISCUITS			
Carr's table water biscuits	Each	14	0.3
Jacob's cream crackers	Each	34	1.1
Nairn's oatcakes	Each	45	2.0
Ryvita crackers, golden rye	Each	27	0.2
Ryvita multigrain crispbread	Each	37	0.6
Ryvita rye crispbread	Each	32	0.2
Ryvita wholegrain crackerbread	Each	20	0.2
Snack-a-Jacks Jumbo, cheese	Each	38	0.3
Tuc snack cracker	Each	24	1.3
CEREAL BARS			
Alpen Fruit & nut bars, milk chocolate	Each	125	3.9
Eat Natural, almond, apricot & yoghurt	Each	228	12
Jordan's Absolute Nut bar	Each	243	18
Jordan's Crunchy bar, honey & almond	Each	139	6.8
Jordan's Frusli bar, raisin & hazelnut	Each	117	3.7
Kellogg's Coco Pops snack bar	Each	85	2.5
Kellogg's Elevenses chocolate chip oat cookies	Each	181	8.0
Kellogg's Frosties snack bar	Each	103	3.0
Kellogg's Nutrigrain, strawberry	Each	133	3.0
Kellogg's Rice Krispies squares, marshmallow	Each	118	3.5
McVitie's Go Ahead Fruit bakes, cherry	Each	131	3.0
McVitie's Go Ahead Yoghurt Breaks, raspberry	Each	72	1.8
Nature Valley Crunchy Granola bars, Canadian maple syrup	Each	191	6.9
Special K Bliss bar, chocolate & raspberry	Each	89	2.0
Special K Mini Breaks	Each	99	2.5

*No information available
Tr trace quantities<0.1g

Saturated fat, g	Carbohydrate, g	Protein, g	Fibre, g
0.1	2.5	0.3	0.1
0.4	5.4	0.8	0.3
0.5	5.7	1.1	1.1
Tr	5.1	0.9	0.5
0.1	6.7	1.1	1.8
Tr	6.7	0.9	1.7
Tr	3.9	0.7	0.6
0.1	8.1	0.9	0.2
1.0	2.6	0.3	0.1
1.7	20	2.1	0.5
8.2	26	2.9	2.9
1.7	16	5.0	2.9
0.9	17	2.5	2.0
0.5	19	1.7	1.4
2.0	14	1.5	0.2
3.0	24	2.5	1.5
2.0	18	2.0	0.3
1.0	26	1.5	1.5
2.0	21	0.8	0.3
1.0	26	1.5	1.5
0.8	13	1.0	0.4
0.8	27	3.4	2.5
1.0	16	0.9	0.9
0.8	17	2.0	0.8

Biscuits (sweet) & bars	Av Portion	Calories	Fat, g
SWEET BISCUITS			
Bourbon Creams	Each	67	3.0
Cadbury Dairy Milk biscuits	Each	75	4.3
Cadbury milk chocolate fingers	Each	30	1.5
Chocolate chip cookies	Each	57	2.6
Chocolate Hobnobs	Each	92	4.5
Custard creams	Each	65	2.7
Digestives	Each	70	3.1
Digestives, light	Each	66	2.4
Fig rolls	Each	63	1.5
Garibaldi	Each	40	0.9
Ginger nuts	Each	53	1.9
Hobnobs	Each	67	3.1
Jaffa cakes	Each	46	1.0
Jam sandwich creams	Each	75	3.4
Jammie dodgers	Each	83	2.8
Milk chocolate digestives	Each	84	4.0
Rich tea	Each	38	1.3
Shortbread fingers	Each	95	5.3
BARS			
Blue Ribband	Each	99	4.9
Club, orange	Each	112	5.9
Fabulous Baking Boys Flapjack	75g bar	346	16
Penguin bar	Each	114	6.1

*No information available
Tr trace quantities<0.1g

Saturated fat, g	Carbohydrate, g	Protein, g	Fibre, g
1.8	9.3	0.8	0.5
2.5	8.4	1.1	0.2
0.6	3.4	0.4	Tr
1.4	7.4	0.7	0.1
2.2	12	1.3	0.9
1.4	8.8	0.7	0.2
0.7	9.3	1.1	0.5
1.1	10	1.1	0.5
0.7	12	0.7	0.6
0.4	7.4	0.5	0.2
0.9	8.3	0.6	0.3
0.7	8.7	1.0	0.8
0.5	8.7	0.6	0.3
2.0	10	0.7	0.3
1.3	13	1.0	0.3
2.1	11	1.2	0.5
0.3	5.9	0.6	0.2
3.4	11	1.2	0.5
3.1	13	0.9	0.2
3.7	13	1.1	0.5
6.9	46	5.1	2.8
3.4	14	1.2	0.5

Bread & bakery	Av Portion	Calories	Fat, g
Bagel, plain	85g	232	1.8
Brioche roll	35g	129	4.6
Brown bread, sliced	1 slice, 40g	85	1.6
Burger bun	85g	224	4.0
Chapatti	55g	111	1.0
Ciabatta bread	1 slice, 30g	92	2.1
Croissant	40g	186	12
Crumpet	40g	77	0.4
French stick	1 slice, 40g	105	1.0
Garlic bread	1 slice, 30g	110	5.0
Hovis Best of Both	1 slice, 40g	86	0.7
Hovis Seed Sensation	1 slice, 44g	122	2.9
Muffin, plain	67g	174	4.7
Naan bread	160g	456	12
Pitta bread, white	60g	153	1.0
Pitta bread, wholemeal	60g	159	0.7
Rye bread	1 slice, 40g	88	1.0
Scotch pancake (Kingsmill)	28g	74	1.2
Soda bread	1 slice, 40g	103	1.0
Tortilla, plain	55g	144	1.0
White bread, sliced	1 slice, 40g	88	1.0
White roll, crusty	50g	131	1.0
White roll, soft	50g	127	1.0
Wholemeal bread, sliced	1 slice, 40g	87	1.0
Wholemeal roll	50g	122	2.0
Wrap	64g	182	3.2

*No information available
Tr trace quantities<0.1g

Saturated fat, g	Carbohydrate, g	Protein, g	Fibre, g
*	49	8.5	2.0
3.0	19	2.8	0.7
*	18	3.2	1.4
0.9	42	7.7	1.3
0.1	24	4.0	*
0.4	16	3.0	0.7
7.0	16	3.2	1.0
Tr	16	2.4	0.9
0.1	22	3.6	1.0
2.9	14	2.3	*
0.2	16	3.6	2.0
0.3	19	4.4	2.3
2.3	26	7.0	1.6
1.6	80	13	3.2
0.1	33	5.5	1.4
*	35	5.5	3.1
0.1	18	3.3	1.8
0.2	14	1.5	0.4
*	22	3.1	0.8
*	33	4.0	1.3
0.1	18	3.2	0.8
0.3	28	4.6	1.2
0.3	26	4.7	1.0
0.2	18	3.2	0.8
0.4	23	5.2	2.2
1.4	32	5.3	2.4

Breakfast cereals	Av Portion	Calories	Fat, g
All Bran, Kellogg's	30g	100	1.1
Alpen high fibre	45g	154	3.2
Alpen original	45g	170	2.6
Bitesize Shredded Wheat	45g	155	1.0
Bran Flakes, Kellogg's	30g	107	0.6
Cheerios	30g	114	3.2
Choco Cornflakes, Kellogg's	30g	117	0.9
Clusters	30g	116	1.5
Coco Pops	30g	116	0.8
Cookie Crisp	30g	115	0.9
Cornflakes, Kellogg's	30g	113	0.3
Country Crisp, raisin	50g	206	6.7
Country Crisp, strawberry	50g	218	8.0
Crunchy Bran, Weetabix	40g	140	1.4
Crunchy Nut Cornflakes, Kellogg's	30g	121	1.5
Curiously Cinnamon	30g	126	3.0
Frosted Wheats	40g	146	0.8
Frosties	30g	113	0.2
Fruit 'n' Fibre	30g	114	1.8
Golden Grahams	30g	115	0.9
Golden Nuggets	30g	113	0.4
Granola, Quaker Oats	50g	205	4.4
Harvest Crunch, fruity raisins	45g	200	6.8
Honey Loops	30g	113	0.9
Honey Nut Shredded Wheat	40g	151	2.6
Hot Oat Crumbly, original	45g	217	9.9

*No information available
Tr trace quantities<0.1g

Saturated fat, g	Carbohydrate, g	Protein, g	Fibre, g
0.2	14	4.2	8.1
0.4	28	3.5	6.3
0.4	30	5.0	3.2
0.2	32	5.4	5.4
0.2	20	3.0	4.5
1.5	23	2.6	2.1
0.5	25	1.5	0.9
0.5	22	2.7	2.2
0.3	26	1.5	0.6
0.3	24	2.0	1.5
0.1	25	2.1	0.9
1.8	33	3.4	2.9
2.3	33	3.9	3.5
0.2	23	4.8	8.0
0.3	25	1.8	0.8
1.1	23	1.5	1.2
0.1	29	4.0	3.6
Tr	26	1.4	0.6
1.1	21	2.4	2.7
0.3	24	2.0	1.4
0.1	25	2.2	1.1
1.4	37	4.3	2.6
0.7	30	3.2	2.9
0.2	23	2.4	2.1
0.9	28	4.4	3.8
5.0	27	3.6	2.7

Breakfast cereals	Av Portion	Calories	Fat, g
Just Right	30g	111	0.6
Krave, chocolate hazelnut	30g	134	4.8
Muesli, Jordan's fruit & nut	45g	216	5.5
Muesli, Jordan's natural	50g	210	4.1
Nesquik	30g	116	1.2
Oat So Simple	27g (1 sachet)	103	2.3
Oatibix	48g (2 biscuits)	189	3.8
Oatibix Bites	40g	158	2.9
Oatibix Flakes	30g	119	2.0
Oats & More, honey	40g	150	2.0
Oats, Quaker	40g	142	3.2
Optivita, raisin	30g	109	1.4
Ready Brek, original	30g	112	2.6
Rice Krispies	30g	115	0.3
Ricicles	30g	115	0.2
Shredded Wheat	45g	153	2.8
Shreddies	40g	148	0.8
Special K	30g	114	0.5
Special K clusters, honey	30g	117	0.9
Special K fruit & nut	30g	114	0.8
Special K strawberry & chocolate	30g	116	0.9
Start	30g	117	1.1
Weetabix	37.5g (2 biscuits)	134	0.8
Weetabix Mini, chocolate chip	40g	155	2.1
Weetos	30g	118	1.5

*No information available
Tr trace quantities<0.1g

Saturated fat, g	Carbohydrate, g	Protein, g	Fibre, g
0.1	24	2.1	1.4
1.8	20	2.4	1.2
2.3	32	7.8	3.2
1.5	35	8.0	4.7
0.5	23	2.3	2.0
0.4	16	3.0	2.5
0.6	31	6.0	3.5
0.4	27	4.2	4.0
0.3	27	2.9	2.2
0.4	29	3.9	2.5
0.6	24	4.4	3.6
0.2	20	2.7	2.4
0.4	17	3.5	2.4
Tr	27	1.4	0.2
Tr	27	1.4	0.2
0.3	31	5.2	5.3
0.2	30	4.0	4.0
0.2	23	4.2	0.8
0.2	24	2.7	1.2
0.1	23	3.6	0.8
0.3	23	3.6	0.9
0.6	24	2.4	1.5
0.2	26	4.3	3.8
1.0	28	3.8	3.8
0.3	23	2.5	1.9

Cakes, pastries & buns	Av Portion	Calories	Fat, g
Battenburg cake	40g slice	149	7.0
Carrot cake	75g slice	269	17
Chocolate cake	75g slice	342	20
Chocolate fudge cake	75g slice	269	11
Chocolate roll	30g each	116	5.0
Cream horn	60g each	261	21
Currant bun	60g each	168	3.0
Custard tart	90g each	249	13
Danish pastry	110g each	376	16
Doughnut, iced	75g each	287	13
Doughnut, jam	75g each	252	11
Éclair	40g each	149	10
Fruit cake	60g slice	223	9.0
Fruit cake, iced	70g slice	245	7.0
Fruit scone	60g each	189	5.0
Gingerbread	50g slice	190	6.0
Hot cross bun	70g each	218	5.0
Iced cup cake	40g each	142	4.0
Jam tart	40g each	153	6.0
Madeira cake	75g slice	283	11
Mince pie	55g each	239	12
Scone, plain	60g each	218	9.0
Sponge cake, cream & jam	60g slice	168	7.0
Sponge cake, jam	60g slice	181	3.0
Swiss roll	30g slice	83	1.0
Teacake	60g each	178	3.0

*No information available
Tr trace quantities<0.1g

Saturated fat, g	Carbohydrate, g	Protein, g	Fibre, g
1.4	21	2.2	0.4
4.1	28	3.2	0.8
*	38	5.6	*
3.4	42	3.9	0.7
2.1	17	1.3	*
10	16	2.3	0.5
1.1	32	4.8	1.3
5.5	29	5.7	1.1
9.4	56	6.4	1.8
*	41	3.6	*
3.2	37	4.3	*
*	15	1.6	0.2
4.1	35	3.1	*
1.2	46	2.5	0.9
1.4	34	3.9	1.2
*	32	2.8	0.6
1.3	41	5.2	1.3
1.3	28	1.5	*
2.7	25	1.3	*
6.3	44	4.1	0.7
*	33	2.3	1.0
2.2	32	4.3	1.1
*	26	2.6	0
1.0	39	2.5	1.1
*	17	2.2	0.2
*	32	4.8	*

Cheese	Av Portion	Calories	Fat, g
Babybel	20g (1 mini)	63	5.0
Blue Stilton	40g	164	14
Brie	40g	137	12
Camembert	40g	116	9.0
Cheddar	40g	166	14
Cheddar, half fat	40g	109	6.0
Cheestrings	21g (1 cheestring)	69	5.0
Cheshire	40g	152	13
Cottage cheese	40g	40	2.0
Cream cheese	30g (1 tbsp)	132	14
Danish blue	40g	137	12
Double Gloucester	40g	162	14
Edam	40g	136	10
Emmental	40g	153	12
Feta	40g	100	8.0
Goat's cheese	40g	128	101
Gouda	40g	151	12
Gruyère	40g	164	13
Mozzarella	40g	103	8.0
Parmesan	10g (1 tbsp)	42	3.0
Philadelphia	30g (1 tbsp)	74	7.0
Philadelphia light	30g (1 tbsp)	47	3.5
Processed cheese	20g (1 slice)	59	5.0
Red Leicester	40g	160	13
Ricotta	40g	58	4.0
Wensleydale	40g	151	13

*No information available
Tr trace quantities<0.1g

Saturated fat, g	Carbohydrate, g	Protein, g	Fibre, g
*	0	4.5	0
9.2	0	9.5	0
7.3	0	8.1	0
5.7	0	8.6	0
8.7	0	10	0
4.0	0	13	0
3.1	0	5.9	0
7.8	0	9.6	0
0.9	1.2	5.0	0
8.9	0	0.9	0
7.7	0	8.2	0
8.5	0	9.8	0
6.3	0	11	0
7.4	0	12	0
5.5	0.6	6.2	0
7.2	0.4	8.4	0
8.1	0	10	0
8.3	0	11	0
5.5	0	7.4	0
1.9	0.1	3.6	0
4.1	0.9	1.7	0.1
2.3	1.2	2.5	0.1
2.9	1.0	3.6	0
8.4	0	9.7	0
2.8	0.8	0.8	0
7.9	0	9.3	0

Confectionery	Av Portion	Calories	Fat, g
Aero, peppermint chunky bar	1 bar	157	8.9
Boiled sweets	25g	82	0
Boost	1 bar	310	17
Bounty twin bar	57g, 1 twin bar	268	14
Bournville plain chocolate	45g, 1 bar	225	12
Buttons, Cadbury's	33g, 1 pack	170	9.6
Celebrations	100g	492	24
Chew sweets	25g	95	1
Chocolate orange, milk chocolate	26g, 3 segments	138	7.8
Chocolate, milk	50g	260	15
Chocolate, plain	50g	255	14
Chocolate, white	50g	265	15
Creme egg	Each	180	6.3
Crunchie	1 bar	185	7.6
Dairy Milk bar	49g, 1 bar	260	15
Dairy Milk bar, fruit & nut	49g, 1 bar	240	13
Double Decker	1 bar	275	11
Dream	1 bar	250	15
Flake	1 bar	170	9.9
Fruit gums	25g	81	0
Fruit pastilles	1 tube	187	0
Fudge	25g	110	3.0
Fudge bar	1 bar	110	3.9
Galaxy	46g, 1 bar	250	15
Jelly Beans	25g	95	Tr
Kit Kat	4 fingers	233	12

*No information available
Tr trace quantities<0.1g

Saturated fat, g	Carbohydrate, g	Protein, g	Fibre, g
5.1	18	1.5	0.3
0	22	0	0
13	35	3.5	0.5
12	33	2.4	1.0
7.5	27	2.1	0.9
6.0	18	2.4	0.2
14	62	5.6	1.2
0.8	22	0.3	0.3
4.6	15	1.9	0.5
9.1	29	3.8	0.4
8.4	32	2.5	1.3
9.2	29	4.0	*
3.9	29	1.6	0.2
4.9	28	1.4	0.5
9.1	28	3.7	0.3
7.1	27	4.1	0.7
7.4	41	2.6	0.8
9.5	27	2.0	0
6.1	18	2.6	0.2
0	20	1.6	*
0	45	2.3	0
2.2	20	0.8	0
2.2	19	0.6	0.1
8.9	26	3.0	0.7
Tr	23	Tr	Tr
7.2	29	2.7	0.9

Confectionery	Av Portion	Calories	Fat, g
Lion bar	1 bar	277	14
Liquorice Allsorts	25g	87	1.0
M&Ms, peanut	45g, 1 bag	228	11
Maltesers	37g, 1 bag	187	9.2
Mars bar	58g, 1 bar	260	9.9
Milk Tray	100g	485	24
Milky Bar	1 bar	136	7.9
Milky Way	22g, 1 bar	98	3.5
Mint imperials	1 sweet	10	-
Peppermints	25g	98	0
Picnic	1 bar	230	11
Polo mints	1 tube	139	0.4
Quality Street	3 sweets	133	5.8
Roses	100g	495	25
Smarties	1 tube	91	3.4
Snickers	58g, 1 bar	296	16
Time Out	1 bar	170	9.7
Toffees	24g, 3 sweets	110	4.3
Twirl	1 bar	230	13
Twix	58g, 2 fingers	286	14
Walnut whip	Each	174	8.9
Wine gums	25g	81	Tr
Wispa	1 bar	215	13
Yorkie, original milk	1 bar	302	17

*No information available
Tr trace quantities<0.1g

Saturated fat, g	Carbohydrate, g	Protein, g	Fibre, g
8.6	26	2.6	1.0
0.9	19	0.9	0.5
4.5	27	4.2	1.2
5.6	23	3.0	0.4
4.8	40	2.5	0.7
13	64	3.9	1.3
4.7	14	1.9	0
1.7	16	0.9	0.1
-	2.4	0	0
0	26	0.1	0
5.1	30	3.5	1.0
0.4	34	Tr	0
3.4	19	1.0	0.4
14	62	4.5	0.6
1.9	14	0.8	0.5
5.5	32	5.5	0.8
6.3	18	2.3	0.4
2.4	18	0.4	0.1
8.2	24	3.3	0.3
8.0	37	2.8	0.8
4.9	22	1.9	0.2
Tr	19	0.9	Tr
8.3	21	2.8	0.3
10	32	3.4	1.0

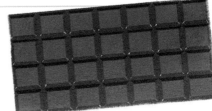

Crisps & snacks	Av Portion	Calories	Fat, g
Burt's potato chips, sea salted	50g	271	14
Doritos, Cool original	35g	175	9.5
Doritos, tangy cheese	35g	175	9.3
Hula hoops	34g	175	9.7
Hula hoops big hoops, chilli	25g	127	6.6
Kallo breadsticks, original	25g	100	1.6
Kallo Torinesi breadsticks, with parmesan	25g	103	2.1
Kettle Chips, Cheddar & red onion	40g	187	10
Kettle Chips, lightly salted	40g	192	10
Kettle Vegetable Chips	25g	121	8.5
Marmite rice cakes	22g	86	0.6
McCoy's ridge cut crisps, flame-grilled steak	50g	259	15
McCoy's ridge cut crisps, Mexican chilli	50g	257	15
McCoy's ridge cut crisps, salt & malt vinegar	50g	258	15
Mini Cheddars	25g	162	7.5
New York Style bagel crisps	50g	232	11
New York Style pitta crisps	50g	242	10
Penn State pretzels, salted	50g	188	0.5
Pringles, original	25g	131	8.4
Pringles, salt & vinegar	25g	129	8.0
Pringles, sour cream & onion	25g	129	8.2
Quavers, cheese	20g	109	6.2
Red Sky crisps, Anglesey sea salt	40g	185	8.7
Red Sky crisps, English Cheddar & red onion	40g	183	8.4
Red Sky crisps, sour cream & green herb	40g	188	9.4

*No information available
Tr trace quantities<0.1g

Saturated fat, g	Carbohydrate, g	Protein, g	Fibre, g
1.5	23	2.6	*
0.9	20	2.6	1.1
1.1	20	2.9	1.1
0.9	21	1.1	0.6
0.6	16	0.9	0.6
0.3	19	2.5	0.3
0.8	18	3.3	0.3
1.2	21	3.0	2.5
1.2	22	2.5	2.0
0.9	9.8	1.4	3.2
0.1	17	3.3	0.8
1.4	27	3.5	2.0
1.4	27	3.5	2.3
1.4	27	3.4	2.0
3.0	13	3.0	0.7
4.5	30	3.6	3.6
2.7	33	5.7	1.7
Tr	9.3	1.3	0.6
1.8	13	1.0	0.7
1.7	13	0.9	0.6
1.8	13	1.0	0.6
0.6	13	0.6	0.2
0.7	24	2.7	2.0
0.7	24	2.8	2.0
1.0	23	2.7	1.9

Crisps & snacks	Av Portion	Calories	Fat, g
Ryvitas Minis, salt & vinegar	30g	94	0.8
Snack-a-Jacks Jumbos, cheese	10g (1 cake)	38	0.3
Snack-a-Jacks, salt & vinegar	22g	89	1.6
Tyrell's crisps, lightly salted	40g	197	10
Tyrell's crisps, mature Cheddar & chives	40g	194	10
Tyrell's crisps, sea salt & black pepper	40g	194	10
Tyrell's crisps, sea salt & cider vinegar	40g	197	9.8
Tyrell's popcorn, sweet & salty	20g	90	4.9
Tyrell's vegetable crisps	25g	184	13
Walkers Baked, cheese & onion	25g	99	2.1
Walkers Baked, ready salted	25g	98	2.0
Walkers Baked, salt & vinegar	25g	98	2.0
Walkers crisps, cheese & onion	34.5g	184	11
Walkers crisps, ready salted	34.5g	185	12
Walkers crisps, salt & vinegar	34.5g	181	11
Walkers crisps, steak & onion	34.5g	183	11
Walkers Lights, sour cream & onion	25g	115	5.3
Walkers Lights, cheese & onion	25g	115	5.3
Walkers Lights, simply salted	25g	115	5.3
Walkers Max, chargrilled steak	50g	262	16
Walkers Max, cheese & onion	50g	264	17
Walkers Max, cheeseburger	50g	266	16
Walkers Sensations, Balsamic vinegar & caramelised onion	35g	170	9.1
Walkers Sensations, lime & coriander poppadoms	35g	168	8.0
Walkers Sensations, Thai sweet chilli	35g	170	9.1
Walkers Sunbites, sea salted	25g	120	5.4
Walkers Sunbites, sour cream	25g	120	5.4

*No information available
Tr trace quantities<0.1g

Saturated fat, g	Carbohydrate, g	Protein, g	Fibre, g
0.1	19	2.0	3.6
0.1	8.1	0.9	0.2
0.1	9.1	0.9	0.2
0.9	24	3.1	1.0
1.1	24	3.4	1.0
1.1	24	3.4	1.0
0.9	24	3.1	1.0
0.6	10	1.3	2.4
1.4	14	2.0	4.8
0.3	18	1.6	1.4
0.3	19	1.5	1.4
0.3	18	1.5	1.3
0.9	17	2.4	1.4
0.9	17	2.0	1.4
0.9	17	2.0	1.4
0.9	17	2.1	1.4
0.5	15	1.8	1.1
0.5	15	1.8	1.1
0.5	15	1.7	1.2
2.1	26	3.6	1.5
2.1	26	3.4	1.5
2.1	26	3.3	1.5
0.9	20	2.1	1.5
0.8	22	2.6	1.6
0.7	20	2.1	1.5
0.6	15	1.8	1.7
0.6	15	1.9	1.7

Eating out	Av Portion	Calories	Fat, g
STARBUCKS			
Almond croissant	Each	433	22
Butter croissant	Each	266	16
Caffe latte, skimmed	Tall	102	0.2
Caffe Americano	Tall	12	0
Caffe latte, semi-skimmed	Tall	148	5.6
Caffe mocha, semi-skimmed, with whipped cream	Tall	266	13
Cappuccino, semi-skimmed	Tall	91	3.4
Cappuccino, skimmed	Tall	64	0.1
Cheese & Marmite panini	Each	382	18
Classic blueberry muffin	Each	481	22
Classic hot chocolate, semi-skimmed, with whipped cream	Tall	261	13
Frapuccino, coffee, semi-skimmed	Tall	170	1.6
Mozzarella & slow roast tomato panini	Each	468	20
Pain au chocolat	Each	269	20
Pain aux raisins	Each	373	19
Roasted chicken & tomato panini	Each	347	8.0
Skinny blueberry muffin	Each	372	5.5
CAFFÉ NERO			
Chicken Caesar wrap	Each	434	23
Chicken salad sandwich	Each	272	4.2
Falafel wrap	Each	434	22
Ham & free-range egg mayonnaise breakfast muffin	Each	314	12
Pesto chicken panini	Each	385	13
Tuna melt panini	Each	389	14
Vine tomato, mozzarella & basil panini	Each	398	17

*No information available
Tr trace quantities<0.1g

Saturated fat, g	Carbohydrate, g	Protein, g	Fibre, g
9.7	52	5.2	1.5
9.3	27	4.1	0.9
0.2	15	9.9	0
0	2.0	0.7	0
3.6	14	9.7	0
7.1	33	10	1.4
2.2	9.0	6.0	0
0.1	9.5	6.1	0
11	35	20	1.4
2.2	256	6.0	2.1
7.1	32	10	1.4
1.0	36	2.8	0.1
8.1	50	20	2.7
9.5	27	3.7	1.7
11	44	5.2	1.5
0.9	51	21	3.1
0.8	73	5.8	3.2
5.0	36	21	1.3
0.6	38	19	3.0
5.3	46	14	2.9
2.1	35	15	2.3
2.5	41	25	2.4
7.2	42	23	2.3
7.5	43	18	2.7

Eating out	Av Portion	Calories	Fat, g
MCDONALD'S			
Big Mac		490	24
Cheeseburger		295	12
Chicken McNuggets	6 pieces	250	14
Filet-o-Fish		350	16
French fries	Medium	330	16
Hamburger		250	8.0
Spicy vegetable wrap		445	16
Sweet chilli crispy chicken wrap		460	18
BURGER KING			
Angus burger		580	31
Chicken Royale		608	32
Fries	Regular	291	12
Hamburger		284	11
Veggie Bean Burger		590	20
Whopper		651	36
KFC			
Fillet burger		449	16
Flamin' wrap		337	16
Fried chicken	3 pieces	735	43
Fried chicken	1 piece	244	15
Fries	Regular	247	12
Hot wings	1 wing	81	5.6
Popcorn chicken	Regular	283	17
Zinger burger		476	19

*No information available
Tr trace quantities<0.1g

Saturated fat, g	Carbohydrate, g	Protein, g	Fibre, g
10	41	28	4
6	31	16	2
2	20	14	1
3	36	15	2
2	42	3	4
3	30	14	2
3	59	10	10
3	53	20	3
9	41	31	2
4	51	25	3
4	39	4	5
4	30	15	1
5	83	18	8
9	51	29	2
2.8	7.7	21	*
3.8	30	18	*
9	23	63	*
2.8	7.7	21	*
1.3	37	3.7	*
0.9	2.9	50	*
1.6	15	18	*
3.1	48	28	*

Eating out	Av Portion	Calories	Fat, g
JD WETHERSPOON			
8oz sirloin steak, chips, peas & tomato		987	60
Breaded scampi, chips & peas		996	49
Chicken Caesar salad		623	41
Classic 6oz beefburger		1064	42
Hand-battered fish, chips & peas		1182	66
Roast of the day: beef		679	18
Roast of the day: half roast chicken		1187	59
Sausages & mash		715	31
Steak & kidney pudding		1143	64
PIZZA HUT			
BBQ American, large pan	1 slice	310	12
BBQ American, regular pan	1 slice	202	8.3
Chicken supreme, large pan	1 slice	279	11
Chicken supreme, regular pan	1 slice	184	7.6
Hawaiian, large pan	1 slice	275	11
Hawaiian, regular pan	1 slice	183	7.7
Margherita, large pan	1 slice	282	13
Margherita, large stuffed crust	1 slice	328	15
Margherita, regular pan	1 slice	188	8.7
Meat feast, large pan	1 slice	316	15
Meat feast, regular pan	1 slice	190	8.5
Veggie supreme, large pan	1 slice	262	11
Veggie supreme, regular pan	1 slice	156	6.2

*No information available
Tr trace quantities<0.1g

Saturated fat, g	Carbohydrate, g	Protein, g	Fibre, g
19	69	57	11
5.4	111	32	12
13	16	47	2.5
12	108	43	8.9
13	97	52	11
5.2	68	62	14
16	67	97	9.6
11	69	39	12
25	110	33	11
4.0	35	16	*
2.7	22	9.8	*
3.5	31	14	*
2.4	20	8.9	*
3.6	32	12	*
2.5	21	8.1	*
4.6	31	11	*
7.4	34	15	*
3.1	20	7.5	*
4.7	31	16	*
2.4	20	8.8	*
3.5	32	9.9	*
1.7	20	5.3	*

Eggs	Av Portion	Calories	Fat, g
Duck eggs, raw	75g (1 egg)	122	9.0
Egg white	32g (1 egg)	12	0
Egg yolk	18g (1 egg)	61	5.0
Eggs, boiled	50g (1 egg)	74	5.0
Eggs, fried	60g (1 egg)	107	8.0
Eggs, poached	50g (1 egg)	74	5.0
Eggs, raw, size 2	61g (1 egg)	87	7.0
Eggs, raw, size 3	57g (1 egg)	82	6.0
Eggs, scrambled with milk	120g (2 eggs)	308	28
Omelette, plain	120g (2 eggs)	234	20
Quail eggs	10g (1 egg)	15	1.0

*No information available
Tr trace quantities<0.1g

Saturated fat, g	Carbohydrate, g	Protein, g	Fibre, g
2.2	0	11	0
0	0	2.9	0
1.6	0	2.9	0
1.5	0	6.3	0
2.4	0	8.2	0
1.5	0	6.3	0
1.8	0	7.6	0
1.7	0	7.1	0
14	0.8	13	0
8.7	0	13	0
0.3	0	1.3	0

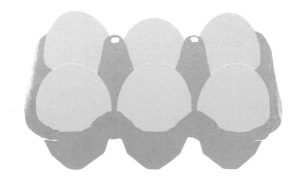

Fats & oils	Av Portion	Calories	Fat, g
FATS			
Anchor spreadable	10g (2 tsp)	72	8.0
Benecol spread	10g (2 tsp)	58	6.3
Bertolli spread	10g (2 tsp)	54	5.9
Butter	10g (2 tsp)	74	8.0
Clover spread	10g (2 tsp)	67	7.5
Flora light spread	10g (2 tsp)	35	3.8
Flora original spread	10g (2 tsp)	53	5.9
Flora Pro-activ spread	10g (2 tsp)	32	3.5
Ghee	10g (2 tsp)	90	10
I Can't Believe it's Not Butter	10g (2 tsp)	62	7.0
Lard	15g (1 tbsp)	134	15
Lurpak spreadable	10g (2 tsp)	73	8.0
Margarine, polyunsaturated	10g (2 tsp)	75	8.0
Pure sunflower spread	10g (2 tsp)	60	6.7
Suet	15g (1 tbsp)	124	13
OILS			
Coconut oil	11g (1 tbsp)	99	11
Corn oil	11g (1 tbsp)	99	11
Frylight sunflower oil spray	0.7g (4 sprays)	4	0.4
Olive oil	11g (1 tbsp)	99	11
Sesame oil	11g (1 tbsp)	99	11
Soya oil	11g (1 tbsp)	99	11
Sunflower oil	11g (1 tbsp)	99	11
Vegetable oil, blended	11g (1 tbsp)	99	11

*No information available
Tr trace quantities<0.1g

Saturated fat, g	Carbohydrate, g	Protein, g	Fibre, g
3.1	0.1	0.1	0
1.5	0.1	Tr	0
1.4	0.1	Tr	0
5.2	0.1	0.1	0
2.7	0.1	0.1	0
0.9	0.3	Tr	0
1.2	Tr	Tr	0
0.9	0.3	Tr	0
6.6	0	0	0
2.4	0.1	0.1	0
6.0	0	0	0
4.0	0.1	0.1	0
1.7	0	0	0
1.5	0	0	0
7.5	1.8	0	0
9.5	0	0	0
1.6	0	0	0
Tr	Tr	Tr	0
2.2	0	0	0
1.6	0	0	0
1.7	0	0	0
1.3	0	0	0
1.3	0	0	0

Fish	Av Portion	Calories	Fat, g
Anchovies, canned in oil, drained	10g (3)	19	1.0
Bass, sea	120g	120	3.0
Bream, sea	120g	115	3.0
Cod, baked	120g	115	1.0
Cod, poached	120g	113	2.0
Cod, smoked, poached	120g	121	1.0
Coley, steamed	120g	126	2.0
Dover sole	140g	125	3.0
Haddock, grilled	120g	125	1.0
Haddock, poached	120g	136	5.0
Haddock, smoked, poached	150g	201	9.0
Halibut, grilled	145g	175	3.0
Halibut, poached	110g	169	6.0
Herring, grilled	110g	199	12
Kipper, baked	130g	267	15
Kipper, grilled	130g	332	25
Lemon sole, grilled	110g	107	2.0
Mackerel, canned in brine, drained	200g	474	36
Mackerel, canned in tomato sauce	125g	258	19
Mackerel, grilled	150g	359	26
Mackerel, smoked	150g	531	46
Monkfish, grilled	120g	115	1.0
Pilchards, canned in tomato sauce	215g (1 tin)	310	17
Plaice, grilled	130g	125	2.0
Pollack, Alaskan	140g	101	1.0
Red snapper, fried	120g	151	4.0

*No information available
Tr trace quantities<0.1g

Saturated fat, g	Carbohydrate, g	Protein, g	Fibre, g
0.2	0	2.5	0
0.5	0	23	0
*	0	21	0
0.4	0	26	0
0.7	0	25	0
0.7	0	26	0
0.2	0	28	0
*	0	25	0
0.2	0	29	0
3.1	1.3	21	0
5.6	1.7	28	0
0.6	0	37	0
3.0	1.2	27	0
3.1	0	22	0
2.3	0	33	0
4.0	0	26	0
0.2	0	22	0
8.0	0	38	0
4.1	1.7	21	0
5.3	0	38	0
9.5	0	28	0
0.1	0	27	0
3.7	2.4	26	0
0.4	0	26	0
0.1	0	23	0
0.8	0	29	0

Fish & seafood	Av Portion	Calories	Fat, g
Salmon, grilled	115g	247	15
Salmon, canned in brined, drained	100g (1 tin)	153	7.0
Salmon, smoked	110g	156	5.0
Sardines, canned in brine, drained	100g (1 tin)	172	10
Sardines, canned in oil, drained	100g (1 tin)	220	14
Sardines, canned in tomato sauce	100g (1 tin)	162	10
Sardines, grilled	40g	78	4.0
Swordfish, grilled	125g	174	6.0
Trout, rainbow, grilled	155g	209	8.0
Tuna	120g	163	6.0
Tuna, canned in brine, drained	100g (1 tin)	99	1.0
Tuna, canned in oil, drained	100g (1 tin)	189	9.0
SEAFOOD			
Clams, canned in brine, drained	50g	39	0.5
Cockles, boiled	25g	13	0.5
Crab, boiled	85g	109	5.0
Lobster, boiled, weighed with shell	250g	93	2.0
Mussels, boiled, weighed with shells	90g	25	1.0
Oysters, weighed with shells	500g	45	1.0
Prawns, boiled	60g	59	1.0
Scallops, steamed	70g	83	1.0
Scampi, in breadcrumbs, fried	170g	403	23
Shrimps, boiled	50g	59	1.0
Squid	140g	113	2.0
Whelks	30g	27	0.5
Winkles	30g	22	0.5

*No information available
Tr trace quantities<0.1g

Saturated fat, g	Carbohydrate, g	Protein, g	Fibre, g
2.9	0	28	0
1.3	0	24	0
0.9	0	28	0
*	0	22	0
2.9	0	23	0
2.8	1.4	17	0
1.2	0	10	0
1.5	0	29	0
1.7	0	33	0
1.4	0	28	0
0.2	0	24	0
1.5	0	27	0
0.1	0.9	8.0	0
0.1	0	3.0	0
0.6	0	17	0
0.3	0	20	0
0.1	0.8	4.1	0
Tr	2.0	7.5	0
0.1	0	9.5	0
0.3	2.4	16	0
2.7	25	16	*
0.2	0	12	0
0.6	1.7	22	0
0.1	0	5.9	0
0.1	0	4.6	0

Fish products & dishes	Av Portion	Calories	Fat, g
FISH PRODUCTS			
Bird's Eye cod fish cakes in crunch crumbs	100g (2 cakes)	187	8.5
Bird's Eye cod fish fingers	84g (3 fingers)	185	7.6
Bird's Eye fish fillets in breadcrumbs	100g (1 fillet)	218	8.2
Bird's Eye omega 3 fish fingers	84g (3 fingers)	185	7.8
Bird's Eye salmon fish fingers	84g (3 fingers)	190	8.0
Bird's Eye Simply fish fillets in batter	100g (1 fillet)	235	13
Jamie Oliver crispy salmon and Pollock fish cakes	100g (2 cakes)	190	8.6
Young's breaded haddock fillets	125g (1 fillet)	234	8.7
Young's fish cakes	106g (2 cakes)	168	6.6
Young's haddock fish fingers	87g (3 fingers)	160	8.0
Young's omega 3 fish fingers	100g (4 fingers)	216	11
Young's Chip Shop large fish fillets	20g (1 fillet)	262	15
Young's cod steaks in butter sauce	140g (1 steak)	107	3.2
Young's cod steaks in parsley sauce	140g (1 steak)	101	2.6
FISH DISHES			
Bird's Eye Baked to Perfection haddock fillets	280g	175	7.8
Bird's Eye Baked to Perfection wild pink salmon fillets	280g	200	12
Young's fish and chips	300g	489	22
Young's original ocean pie	400g	440	16

*No information available
Tr trace quantities<0.1g

Saturated fat, g	Carbohydrate, g	Protein, g	Fibre, g
1.1	16	12	1.0
0.8	18	11	0.8
1.1	24	12	1.2
0.9	18	10	0.8
0.9	18	11	0.8
1.7	19	11	0.7
0.9	17	9.9	1.7
1.0	22	17	1.5
2.0	19	9.0	1.4
0.9	11	12	1.2
1.2	17	13	0.8
2.8	18	13	1.1
2.2	5.8	14	0.6
1.7	5.9	13	0.6
5.0	2.5	24	0.2
6.5	0.6	23	tr
2.1	53	20	4.2
7.7	47	24	4.8

Fruit	Av Portion	Calories	Fat, g
Apples, cooking, peeled	130g (one)	46	Tr
Apples, eating	100g (one)	47	Tr
Apricots, canned in juice	80g	27	Tr
Apricots, canned in syrup	80g	50	Tr
Apricots, fresh	40g (one)	12	Tr
Apricots, dried, ready-to-eat	40g (3)	63	Tr
Avocado	145g (one)	276	28
Bananas	100g (one)	95	0.3
Blackberries	80g	20	Tr
Blackcurrants	80g	22	Tr
Cherries, canned in syrup	80g	57	Tr
Cherries, glacé	25g (1 tbsp)	63	Tr
Cherries, fresh	80g	38	Tr
Clementines	60g (one)	22	Tr
Cranberries	80g	12	Tr
Dates, dried	25g (1 tbsp)	68	Tr
Dates, fresh	25g (3)	31	Tr
Dried mixed fruit	25g (1 handful)	67	Tr
Figs, fresh	55g (one)	24	Tr
Figs, dried	25g (3)	52	Tr
Fruit cocktail, canned in juice	80g	23	Tr
Gooseberries	80g	32	Tr
Grapefruit, canned in juice	80g	24	Tr
Grapefruit, fresh	80g (half)	24	Tr
Grapes	80g	48	Tr
Guava, canned in syrup	80g	48	Tr

*No information available
Tr trace quantities<0.1g

Saturated fat, g	Carbohydrate, g	Protein, g	Fibre, g
0	12	0.4	2.1
0	12	0.4	1.8
0	6.7	0.4	0.7
0	13	0.3	0.7
0	2.9	0.4	0.7
0	15	1.6	2.5
5.9	28	28	49
0	23	1.2	1.1
0	4.1	0.7	2.5
0	5.3	0.7	2.9
0	15	0.4	0.5
0	17	0.1	0.2
0	9.2	0.7	0.7
0	5.2	0.5	0.7
0	2.7	0.3	2.4
0	17	0.8	1.0
0	7.8	0.4	0.4
0	17	0.6	0.6
0	5.2	0.7	0.9
0	12	0.8	1.7
0	5.8	0.3	0.8
0	7.4	0.6	1.9
0	5.8	0.5	0.3
0	5.4	0.6	1.0
0	12	0.3	0.6
0	13	0.3	2.4

Fruit	Av Portion	Calories	Fat, g
Guava	150g (one)	39	0.8
Kiwi fruit	60g (one)	29	Tr
Lemon juice	10g (half)	1	0
Lime juice	10g (half)	1	0
Lychees, canned in syrup	80g	54	Tr
Lychees, fresh	15g (one)	9	Tr
Mandarin oranges, canned in juice	80g	26	Tr
Mandarin oranges, canned in syrup	80g	42	Tr
Mangoes	150g (one)	86	Tr
Melon, cantaloupe	150g (1 slice)	29	Tr
Melon, galia	150g (1 slice)	36	Tr
Melon, honeydew	150g (1 slice)	42	Tr
Melon, watermelon	200g (1 slice)	62	0.3
Nectarines	150g (one)	60	Tr
Olives, in brine	25g (1 handful)	26	3.0
Oranges	160g (one)	59	Tr
Passion fruit	15g (one)	5	Tr
Papaya	140g (one)	50	Tr
Peaches	110g (one)	36	tr
Peaches, canned in juice	80g	31	tr
Peaches, canned in syrup	80g	44	Tr
Pears	160g (one)	64	Tr
Pears, canned in juice	80g	26	Tr
Pears, canned in syrup	80g	40	Tr
Pineapple, canned in juice	80g	38	Tr
Pineapple, canned in syrup	80g	51	Tr
Pineapple	80g (2 rings)	33	Tr

*No information available
Tr trace quantities<0.1g

Saturated fat, g	Carbohydrate, g	Protein, g	Fibre, g
Tr	7.5	1.2	5.6
0	6.4	0.7	1.1
0	0.2	0	0
0	0.2	0	0
0	14	0.3	0.4
0	2.1	0.1	0.1
0	6.2	0.6	0.2
0	11	0.4	0.2
0	21	1.0	3.9
0	6.3	0.9	1.5
0	8.4	0.8	0.6
0	9.9	0.9	0.9
Tr	14	1.0	0.2
0	14	2.1	1.8
0.4	0	0.2	0.7
0	14	1.8	2.7
0	0.9	0.4	0.5
0	12	0.7	3.1
0	8.4	1.1	1.6
0	7.8	0.5	0.6
0	11	0.4	0.7
0	16	0.5	3.5
0	6.8	0.2	1.1
0	11	0.2	0.9
0	9.8	0.2	0.4
0	13	0.4	0.6
0	8.1	0.3	1.0

Fruit	Av Portion	Calories	Fat, g
Plums	55g (one)	20	Tr
Plums, canned in syrup	80g	47	Tr
Pomegranate	100g (one)	51	Tr
Prunes, canned in juice	80g	64	Tr
Prunes, canned in syrup	80g	72	Tr
Prunes, ready-to-eat	40g (8)	56	Tr
Raisins	25g (1 handful)	68	Tr
Raspberries, canned in syrup	80g	70	Tr
Raspberries	80g	20	Tr
Redcurrants	80g	17	Tr
Rhubarb, canned in syrup	80g	25	Tr
Rhubarb	80g	6	Tr
Satsumas	60g (one)	22	Tr
Strawberries, canned in syrup	80g	52	Tr
Strawberries	80g	22	Tr
Sultanas	25g (1 handful)	69	Tr
Tangerines	60g (one)	21	Tr

*No information available
Tr trace quantities<0.1g

Saturated fat, g	Carbohydrate, g	Protein, g	Fibre, g
0	4.8	0.3	0.9
0	12	0.2	0.6
0	12	1.3	3.4
0	16	0.6	2.0
0	18	0.4	2.2
0	14	1.0	2.3
0	17	0.5	0.5
0	18	0.5	1.2
0	3.7	1.1	2.0
0	3.5	0.9	2.7
0	6.1	0.4	0.6
0	0.6	0.7	1.1
0	5.1	0.5	0.8
0	14	0.4	0.6
0	4.8	0.6	0.9
0	17	0.7	0.5
0	4.8	0.5	0.8

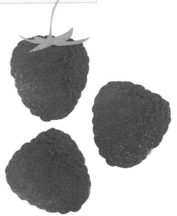

Ice cream	Av Portion	Calories	Fat, g
Dairy ice cream, flavoured	75g, 2 scoops	134	6.0
Dairy ice cream, vanilla	75g, 2 scoops	133	7.0
Ice cream cone	Each, 75g	140	6.0
Non-dairy ice cream, flavoured	75g 2 scoops	125	6.0
Non-dairy ice cream, vanilla	75g 2 scoops	115	6.0
Sorbet, fruit	75g, 2 scoops	73	0
Ben & Jerry's Caramel Chew Chew ice cream	100ml, 2 scoops	240	14
Ben & Jerry's Cherry Garcia frozen yoghurt	100ml, 2 scoops	140	2.5
Ben & Jerry's Chocolate Fudge Brownie frozen yoghurt	100ml, 2 scoops	150	2
Ben & Jerry's Chocolate Fudge Brownie ice cream	100ml, 2 scoops	210	10
Ben & Jerry's Cookie Dough ice cream	100ml, 2 scoops	210	12
Ben & Jerry's Phish Food ice cream	100ml, 2 scoops	230	11
Cadbury's Dairy Milk ice cream bar	100ml, 1 bar	235	15
Carte d'Or Chocolate Inspiration ice cream	100ml, 2 scoops	110	5.0
Carte d'Or Light Vanilla ice cream	100ml, 2 scoops	70	2.0
Carte d'Or Rum & Raisin ice cream	100ml, 2 scoops	100	4.0
Carte d'Or Vanilla ice cream	100ml, 2 scoops	100	4.5
Cornetto Classico	90ml, 1 cone	180	10
Cornetto strawberry	90ml, 1 cone	140	5.0
Del Monte Raspberry Iced Smoothie	90ml, 1 stick	85	Tr
Green & Black's vanilla ice cream	145ml, 3 scoops	219	13
Green & Black's chocolate ice cream	145ml, 3 scoops	248	14
Haagan Dazs Cookies & Cream ice cream	100ml, 1 mini tub	225	14
Haagan Dazs Pralines & Cream ice cream	100ml, 1 mini tub	245	15
Haagan Dazs Strawberry Cheesecake ice cream	100ml, 1 mini tub	236	14

*No information available
Tr trace quantities<0.1g

Saturated fat, g	Carbohydrate, g	Protein, g	Fibre, g
3.9	19	2.6	0
4.6	15	2.7	0
*	19	2.6	0
2.8	17	2.3	0
3.6	14	2.3	0
0	19	0.2	0
9	26	3.5	0.5
2	26	3.5	0.6
1	29	4.5	1
7	25	4	1.5
7	23	3	0.5
8	30	3	1.5
*	25	3.0	*
*	15	2.0	*
2.0	11	1.0	2.0
*	12	1.5	*
*	14	1.5	*
8.0	20	2.5	0.9
4.0	23	1.5	0.6
Tr	21	0.3	0.7
8.0	20	4.5	0.1
8.7	25	5.0	1.1
*	20	3.7	*
*	25	3.6	*
*	25	3.3	*

Ice cream	Av Portion	Calories	Fat, g
Haagan Dazs vanilla ice cream	100ml, 1 mini tub	225	15
Kelly's Cornish clotted vanilla ice cream	125ml, 2 scoops	135	8.9
Kelly's Cornish strawberries & Cream	125ml, 2 scoops	125	5.9
Magnum classic	120ml, 1 stick	260	16
Magnum gold	120ml, 1 stick	280	18
Magnum white	120ml, 1 stick	270	16
Mars ice cream bar	51ml, 1 bar	143	8.3
Nestlé Fab	59ml, 1 stick	90	3.2
Skinny Cow mint double choc ice cream bar	100ml, 1 stick	94	1.9
Skinny Cow triple choc brownie	100ml, 1 stick	93	1.7
Solero fruit ice, orange	55ml, 1 stick	65	Tr
Strawberry Split	73ml, 1 stick	67	1.8
Wall's Classics Cornish vanilla	100ml, 2 scoops	75	3.0
Wall's Soft Scoop vanilla ice cream	100ml, 2 scoops	85	4.0

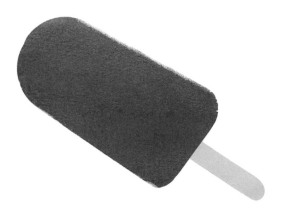

*No information available
Tr trace quantities<0.1g

Saturated fat, g	Carbohydrate, g	Protein, g	Fibre, g
*	18	3.8	*
5.7	12	1.7	0.1
5.2	10	1.9	Tr
12	25	3.0	1.5
14	26	3.0	0.5
12	26	3.5	0.3
*	15	1.8	*
1.4	15	0.3	0.3
1.2	15	2.4	3.0
1.0	16	2.3	3.4
Tr	15	Tr	Tr
1.1	12	0.7	0.2
2.0	11	1.5	0.5
2.0	10	1.5	0.5

Lamb	Av Portion	Calories	Fat, g
Neck cutlets, grilled, trimmed	90g	103	6.0
Neck cutlets, grilled	90g	233	19
Neck fillet, grilled, trimmed	90g	256	17
Neck fillet, grilled	90g	272	20
Chump chops, fried, trimmed	70g	149	8.0
Chump chops, fried	70g	216	16
Leg chops, grilled	70g	155	8.0
Leg joint, roasted, trimmed	90g	189	9.0
Leg joint, roasted	90g	212	12
Leg steaks, grilled trimmed	90g	178	8.0
Leg steaks, grilled	90g	208	12
Loin chops, grilled, trimmed	120g	156	8.0
Loin chops, grilled	120g	296	21
Loin chops, roasted, trimmed	70g	180	9.0
Loin chops, roasted	120g	379	25
Loin joint, roasted, trimmed	90g	188	10
Loin joint, roasted	90g	273	20
Shoulder joint, roasted, trimmed	90g	212	12
Shoulder joint, roasted	90g	254	18
Mince	100g	208	12
Rack of lamb, roasted, trimmed	90g	203	12
Rack of lamb, roasted	90g	327	27

*No information available
Tr trace quantities<0.1g

Saturated fat, g	Carbohydrate, g	Protein, g	Fibre, g
2.8	0	12	0
9.4	0	16	0
7.8	0	25	0
9.3	0	23	0
3.5	0	20	0
7.6	0	17	0
3.5	0	20	0
3.1	0	28	0
4.2	0	27	0
3.2	0	26	0
5.0	0	25	0
3.6	0	21	0
10	0	26	0
4.3	0	24	0
14	0	27	0
4.4	0	25	0
9.5	0	22	0
5.6	0	26	0
8.4	0	23	0
5.8	0	24	0
5.6	0	24	0
13	0	21	0

Milk	Av Portion	Calories	Fat, g
Alpro soya milk alternative, original	100ml	43	1.9
Channel Island milk, whole	100ml	78	5.0
Coconut milk, Amoy	100ml	165	17
Coconut milk, reduced fat, Amoy	100ml	110	11
Condensed milk, skimmed, sweetened	100ml	267	0.2
Condensed milk, whole, sweetened	100ml	333	10
EcoMil Almond organic milk alternative	100ml	46	2.1
Evaporated milk	100ml	151	9.0
Evaporated milk, light	100ml	123	4.0
Flavoured milk	100ml	64	2.0
Goat's milk	100ml	64	4.0
Hot chocolate, made with semi-skimmed milk	100ml	73	2.0
Lactofree, semi-skimmed	100ml	40	1.7
Oatly organic oat drink	100ml	35	0.7
Rice Dream organic milk alternative	100ml	4	1.0
Semi-skimmed milk	100ml	46	2.0
Skimmed milk	100ml	34	0.1
Whole milk	100ml	66	4.0

*No information available
Tr trace quantities<0.1g

Saturated fat, g	Carbohydrate, g	Protein, g	Fibre, g
0.3	2.9	3.3	0.6
3.3	4.8	3.6	0
14	2.0	1.0	1.0
9.0	2.0	1.0	1.0
0.1	60	10	0
6.3	56	8.5	0
0.2	5.4	0.9	0.8
5.9	8.5	8.4	0
2.7	13	9.2	0
1.0	9.6	3.6	0
2.4	4.4	3.1	0
1.3	11	3.6	0
1.1	2.6	3.2	0
0.1	6.5	1.0	0.8
0.1	9.4	0.1	0.1
1.1	4.7	3.5	0
Tr	4.8	3.5	0
2.5	4.6	3.3	0

Offal	Av Portion	Calories	Fat, g
Kidneys, lambs, fried	75g	141	8.0
Kidneys, pigs, stewed	75g	115	5.0
Liver, calves, fried	90g	158	9.0
Livers, chicken, fried	90g	152	8.0
Liver, lambs, fried	90g	213	12

*No information available
Tr trace quantities<0.1g

Saturated fat, g	Carbohydrate, g	Protein, g	Fibre, g
*	0	18	0
1.5	0	18	0
*	0	20	0
*	0	20	0
*	0	27	0

Pasta & pasta dishes	Av Portion	Calories	Fat, g
PASTA			
Egg noodles, uncooked	75g	293	6.0
Lasagne sheets, uncooked	75g	260	2.0
Macaroni, uncooked	75g	261	1.0
Noodles, uncooked	75g	291	5.0
Penne, fresh, uncooked	125g	343	4.0
Spaghetti, fresh, uncooked	125g	350	2.9
Spaghetti, uncooked	75g	257	1.0
Spaghetti, wholemeal, uncooked	75g	243	2.0
Tagliatelle, fresh, uncooked	125g	334	3.1
PASTA DISHES: WAITROSE			
Beef cannelloni	400g	458	22
Beef & red wine ravioli	125g	294	9.6
Cheese, tomato & basil ravioli	125g	276	8.4
Lasagne with beef	400g	433	20
Ricotta & spinach tortelloni	125g	298	7.6
Spaghetti & meatballs	400g	499	27
Spaghetti Bolognese	400g	389	9.6
Spaghetti carbonara	400g	680	35
Spinach & ricotta cannelloni	400g	476	22
Vegetable lasagne	400g	453	27

*No information available
Tr trace quantities<0.1g

Saturated fat, g	Carbohydrate, g	Protein, g	Fibre, g
1.7	54	9.1	2.2
*	56	8.9	2.3
0.2	57	9.0	2.3
*	57	8.8	2.2
1.0	60	16	3.1
0.9	67	13	3.1
0.2	56	9.0	2.2
0.3	50	10	6.3
0.9	67	13	3.1
13	37	27	4.2
3.6	38	14	3.5
4.4	40	12	0.5
10	38	25	4.4
4.4	45	13	3.0
5.7	47	18	4.3
4.2	52	24	4.8
16	60	32	4.0
13	35	18	3.9
10	39	13	4.8

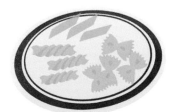

Pasta & pasta dishes	Av Portion	Calories	Fat, g
PASTA DISHES: TESCO			
Cannelloni, Finest	360g	600	20
Chicken & ham pasta bake	400g	595	18
Lasagne al forno, Finest	400g	645	36
Roasted pepper & spinach lasagne	350g	400	22
Spaghetti Bolognese, Finest	450g	705	31
Tuna & pasta bake	400g	535	22
TINNED PASTA DISHES: HEINZ			
Macaroni cheese	200g	174	5.9
Ravioli in tomato sauce	205g	155	3.3
Spaghetti hoops in tomato sauce	200g	109	0.4
Spaghetti in tomato sauce	200g	120	0.5
PASTA DISHES: SAINSBURY'S			
Beef lasagne	400g	609	32
Chicken & bacon pasta bake	400g	648	33
Spaghetti Bolognese	400g	625	28
Spaghetti carbonara	400g	625	29
Spaghetti & meatballs	400g	458	19
Tomato & mozzarella pasta bake	400g	495	14
Vegetable lasagne	400g	456	23
PASTA DISHES: ASDA			
Beef lasagne	400g	476	23
Bolognese pasta bake	400g	630	24
Chilli pasta bake	400g	630	20
Roasted vegetable lasagne	400g	443	20
Spinach & ricotta cannelloni	400g	595	31

*No information available
Tr trace quantities<0.1g

Saturated fat, g	Carbohydrate, g	Protein, g	Fibre, g
12	70	28	11
4.4	78	27	4.4
14	46	35	6.4
10	37	8.8	6.0
11	65	43	6.3
11	50	32	4.8
2.1	23	7.7	0.6
1.2	26	4.9	1.8
Tr	23	3.5	1.2
Tr	25	3.5	4.8
16	53	28	6.6
16	54	31	4.1
11	64	28	6.7
15	68	21	5.2
6.3	43	25	5.8
5.4	71	19	6.0
11	47	11	7.6
11	34	30	5.6
17	70	30	6.0
11	83	28	4.0
9.6	46	16	4.8
19	55	19	7.3

Pastry & savoury pies	Av Portion	Calories	Fat, g
PASTRY			
All butter puff pastry, uncooked (Jus rol)	50g	196	13
Filo pastry, (Jus rol)	50g	117	1.4
Puff pastry, uncooked (Jus rol)	50g	214	13
Shortcrust pastry, uncooked (Jus rol)	50g	229	15
SAVOURY PIES			
Beef pie	150g	449	29
Chicken pie	130g	374	23
Cornish pasty	155g	414	25
Ginsters Cheese & onion slice	180g	500	34
Ginsters Cornish pasty	227g	549	32
Ginsters large sausage roll	140g	499	38
Ginsters pepper steak slice	180g	455	27
Pork & egg pie	60g	178	13
Pork pie, mini	50g	196	14
Pukka Pies all steak pie	230g	538	33
Pukka Pies chicken & mushroom pie	230g	475	29
Pukka Pies steak & kidney pie	230g	488	26
Quiche lorraine, home-made	140g	501	36
Sausage rolls	60g	230	17
Steak & kidney pie, home-made	120g	406	26
Tesco bacon & leek quiche	100g (¼ quiche)	230	15
Tesco cheese & onion quiche	100g (¼ quiche)	265	17
Tesco quiche lorraine	100g (¼ quiche)	175	7.7

*No information available
Tr trace quantities<0.1g

Saturated fat, g	Carbohydrate, g	Protein, g	Fibre, g
9.2	17	2.8	0.7
0.2	26	4.0	1.1
6.9	15	2.5	0.7
5.6	19	3.2	1.1
13	33	11	*
9.1	32	12	1.0
9.1	39	10	1.4
18	35	14	5.2
15	53	12	7.1
16	27	13	2.9
13	38	15	2.9
4.4	10	6.3	*
5.7	13	5.3	0.5
16	37	23	3.7
11	36	17	8.0
12	41	21	8.2
15	27	19	1.0
6.7	15	5.9	0.6
9.7	27	16	1.1
6.5	16	6.5	3.2
7.9	17	8.8	2.5
3.2	15	11	3.8

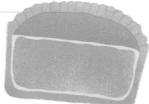

Pizza	Av Portion	Calories	Fat, g
PIZZA EXPRESS			
8in American pizza	½ pizza, 128g	303	11
8in La Reine pizza	½ pizza, 142g	307	9.8
8in Lighter Gustosa	½ pizza, 125g	220	3.9
8in Lighter Vitabella	½ pizza, 125g	215	3.3
8in Margherita pizza	½ pizza, 125g	287	8.5
8in Pollo pesto pizza	½ pizza, 135g	293	5.5
8in Sloppy Guiseppe pizza	½ pizza, 153g	306	10
12in Margherita pizza	⅓ pizza, 164g	374	12
CHICAGO TOWN			
Deep dish ham & pineapple	1 pizza, 170g	398	15
Deep dish meat combo	1 pizza, 170g	434	19
Takeaway four cheese stuffed crust	¼ pizza, 157g	392	15
Takeaway pepperoni stuffed crust pizza	¼ pizza, 161g	428	18
GOODFELLA'S			
Deep Loaded cheese	½ pizza, 209g	526	17
Deep pan pepperoni	½ pizza, 210g	538	20
Flatbread pepperoni speciale	½ pizza, 207g	494	19
Flatbread sweet chilli chicken	½ pizza, 207g	530	18
Stonebaked thin crust roast chicken	½ pizza, 183g	442	17
Stonebaked thin crust vegetable & pesto	½ pizza, 200g	382	13
DR OETKER			
Ristorante Hawaii	½ pizza, 178g	382	15
Ristorante pollo	½ pizza, 178g	378	16
Ristorante quattro formaggi	½ pizza, 165g	431	23
Ristorante speciale	½ pizza, 165g	414	21

*No information available
Tr trace quantities<0.1g

Saturated fat, g	Carbohydrate, g	Protein, g	Fibre, g
5.0	39	13	2.8
3.9	42	13	3.7
1.6	35	12	4.6
2.1	39	10	3.3
1.5	40	13	3.3
2.4	46	15	3.0
4.6	40	13	4.6
6.1	51	17	4.4
7	50	16	2.5
8	49	18	2.5
8.4	47	18	3.2
8.9	47	19	3.2
10	68	25	4.7
8.2	67	23	4.2
8.0	58	20	3.6
7.2	63	26	3.8
6.4	47	26	3.6
6.4	50	16	3.6
5.0	45	15	3.0
5.5	42	15	3.2
10	40	18	2.6
7.6	38	18	3.0

Poultry & game	Av Portion	Calories	Fat, g
CHICKEN			
Breast, grilled, skinned	130g	191	4.0
Breast, grilled, with skin	130g	225	8.0
Chicken curry	350g	522	31
Chicken fricassée	200g	214	12
Chicken goujons	90g	249	13
Chicken Kiev	170g	456	29
Chicken korma	350g	455	20
Chicken pie	130g	374	23
Chicken roll	12g	16	1.0
Chicken slices	40g	46g	1.0
Coronation chicken	200g	728	63
Drumsticks, roasted	90g	104	5.0
Drumsticks, roasted, skinned	47g	71	2.0
Leg quarter, casseroled	146g	317	20
Leg quarter, casseroled, skinned	146g	257	12
Leg quarter, roasted	146g	345	25
Leg quarter, roasted, skinned	146g	134	5.0
Thighs, casseroled	45g	105	7.0
Thighs, casseroled, skinned	45g	81	4.0
Whole, roasted	100g	218	13
Wing quarter, casseroled	150g	315	19
Wing quarter, casseroled, skinned	150g	246	9.0

*No information available
Tr trace quantities<0.1g

Saturated fat, g	Carbohydrate, g	Protein, g	Fibre, g
1.2	0	39	0
1.2	0	38	0
14	19	42	4.5
4.8	5.2	21	1.0
3.6	18	18	0.6
12	19	32	1.0
6.0	16	53	1.4
9.1	32	12	1.0
0.2	0.6	2.1	0
0.2	0.8	9.3	0
11	6.4	33	*
1.4	0	15	0
0.7	0	13	0
5.5	0	33	0
3.4	0	37	0
6.7	0	31	0
1.5	0	23	0
2.0	0	10	0
1.1	0	12	0
3.4	0	26	0
5.3	0	37	0
2.6	0	40	0

Poultry & game	Av Portion	Calories	Fat, g
TURKEY			
Breast, grilled, skinned	100g	155	2.0
Dark meat, roasted	90g	159	6.0
Drumsticks, roasted	45g	84	4.0
Light meat, roasted	90g	138	2.0
Mince, stewed	100g	176	7.0
Roast turkey	90g	154	6.0
Thighs, casseroled, skinned	50g	91	4.0
Turkey slices	23g	26	0.5
Duck, roasted	185g	783	70
Duck, roasted, skinned	185g	361	19
Goose, roasted	185g	557	39
Goose, roasted, skinned	185g	590	41
Pheasant, roasted, skinned	160g	352	19
Pigeon, roasted, skinned	115g	215	9.0
Rabbit, stewed, skinned	160g	182	5.0
Venison, roasted	120g	198	3.0

*No information available
Tr trace quantities<0.1g

Saturated fat, g	Carbohydrate, g	Protein, g	Fibre, g
0.6	0	35	0
1.8	0	27	0
1.2	0	12	0
0.6	0	30	0
2.0	0	29	0
1.9	0	25	0
1.3	0	28	0
0.1	0	5.3	0
21	0	37	0
6.1	0	47	0
12	0	51	0
*	0	54	0
6.6	0	45	0
*	0	33	0
2.7	0	34	0
*	0	43	0

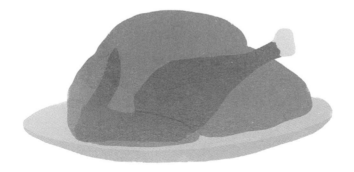

Puddings	Av Portion	Calories	Fat, g
Apple crumble	150g	311	10
Apple pie	110g slice	293	15
Bakewell tart	120g slice	547	22
Blancmange	150g	171	6.0
Bread & butter pudding	150g	240	12
Cheesecake	100g slice	426	36
Chocolate mousse	60g	89	4.0
Christmas pudding	100g	329	12
Crème caramel	100g	102	2.0
Fruit crumble	150g	329	12
Fruit mousse	60g	86	4.0
Fruit pie	110g slice	288	15
Fruit pie, individual	60g each	214	8.0
Jelly	125g	76	0
Lemon meringue pie	80g slice	201	7.0
Pancakes	60g each	181	10
Pavlova	80g	230	11
Profiteroles	90g	311	23
Rice pudding, canned	125g	106	2.0
Rice pudding, canned, low fat	125g	89	1.0
Sponge pudding	110g	374	18
Spotted dick	110g	360	18
Treacle tart	90g slice	341	13
Trifle	150g	249	12

*No information available
Tr trace quantities<0.1g

Saturated fat, g	Carbohydrate, g	Protein, g	Fibre, g
*	55	2.7	2.4
*	39	3.2	1.9
*	52	7.6	2.3
3.4	27	4.6	0
*	26	9.3	0.5
19	25	3.7	0.4
2.0	12	2.4	*
6.1	56	3.0	1.7
0.9	21	3.0	*
6.0	54	3.6	1.9
2.5	11	2.7	*
4.6	37	3.4	1.9
3.2	34	2.6	*
0	19	1.5	0
2.5	35	2.3	0.6
4.2	21	3.6	0.5
5.8	34	2.2	0.2
13	22	5.0	*
0.9	20	4.1	0.1
0.6	17	4.4	0.1
5.6	50	6.4	1.2
*	47	4.6	1.1
3.9	57	3.5	1.0
3.6	32	3.9	0.6

Rice, noodles & rice dishes	Av Portion	Calories	Fat, g
RICE & NOODLES			
Arborio rice, uncooked	60g	213	0.6
Basmati rice, uncooked	60g	215	0.8
Egg noodles, uncooked	60g	235	5.0
Noodles, uncooked	60g	233	4.0
Rice noodles, uncooked	60g	216	Tr
White rice, uncooked	60g	217	0.5
Wholegrain rice, uncooked	60g	214	1.7
RICE DISHES			
Gallo Risotto Pronto, four cheese, uncooked	100g	347	3.0
Gallo Risotto Pronto, porcini mushroom, uncooked	100g	341	1.0
Sainsbury's lemon, thyme & chicken risotto	400g	514	20
Sainsbury's mushroom risotto	400g	502	22
Sainsbury's paella	400g	498	11
Tesco Cook Pot chicken & mushroom risotto	362g	650	26
Tesco Finest mushroom risotto	400g	550	27
Tesco Finest paella	475g	645	24
Tesco vegetable paella	200g	210	8.4
Uncle Ben's chicken and mushroom risotto	125g	223	3.9
Uncle Ben's grilled Mediterranean vegetable risotto	125g	206	3.0
Uncle Ben's tomato & Italian herb risotto	125g	224	5.1
Waitrose Italian bacon & pea risotto	350g	558	32
Waitrose Italian roast mushroom risotto	350g	434	16
Waitrose Menu for One prawn risotto	400g	497	20
Waitrose Menu for Two paella	350g	484	17

*No information available
Tr trace quantities<0.1g

Saturated fat, g	Carbohydrate, g	Protein, g	Fibre, g
Tr	47	4.1	0.3
0.1	48	4.4	*
1.4	43	7.3	1.7
*	46	7.0	1.7
Tr	49	2.9	*
0.1	52	3.9	0.3
0.4	49	4.0	1.1
*	72	8.0	*
*	75	8.0	*
10	43	39	7.5
11	65	8.9	2.3
2.1	69	31	5.6
12	66	36	2.9
14	55	16	9.6
4.7	81	23	6.6
1.2	30	4.6	4.2
0.8	41	5.8	1.1
0.6	39	4.8	1.5
1.6	39	4.6	1.6
13	50	16	3.3
8.7	61	9.8	2.4
11	59	19	1.4
5.0	57	3.8	4.8

Salads	Av Portion	Calories	Fat, g
BAGGED SALADS			
Baby leaf salad	100g	19	0.6
Baby spinach	100g	25	0.8
Caesar salad	100g	150	13
Lamb's lettuce	100g	15	0.5
Pea shoots	100g	19	0.6
Rocket	100g	22	0.3
Watercress	100g	22	1.0
Watercress, rocket & spinach salad	100g	21	0.8
WAITROSE			
Chicken Caesar salad	250g (1 pack)	378	25
Couscous & roasted vegetable salad	200g (1 pack)	316	10
Four bean & buckwheat salad	220g (1 pack)	257	6.2
Fruity Moroccan couscous salad	235g (1 pack)	364	8.5
Pesto & spinach pasta salad	190g (1 pack)	365	18
Pesto, spinach & pinenut pasta salad	165g (1 pack)	339	17
Tomato, basil & chicken pasta salad	205g (1 pack)	310	25
Tuna niçoise salad	330g (1 pack)	343	22
SAINSBURY'S			
Coronation wild rice salad	300g (1 pack)	456	18
Giant couscous & feta salad	220g (1 pack)	360	17
Large salad bowl	80g (1 pack)	15	0.2
Moroccan couscous salad	200g (1 pack)	364	7.2
Rainbow salad	240g (1 pack)	286	6.8

*No information available
Tr trace quantities<0.1g

Saturated fat, g	Carbohydrate, g	Protein, g	Fibre, g
0.1	1.7	1.7	1.9
0.1	1.6	2.8	2.1
2.6	7.0	4.9	1.1
0.1	1.7	0.8	0.9
0.1	0.2	3.1	2.0
0.1	0.9	2.9	2.1
0.3	0.4	3.0	1.5
0.2	1.2	2.2	1.5
5.0	15	23	2.3
1.2	46	11	2.6
0.7	40	11	11
0.9	60	12	5.6
3.4	40	11	2.7
2.3	37	6.9	2.3
3.5	37	17	2.3
3.3	17	18	3.0
3.6	66	7.2	3.0
3.8	36	12	9.6
0.1	2.2	0.9	1.1
0.8	60	8.8	11
0.0	56	12	5.6

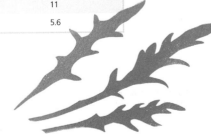

Salads	Av Portion	Calories	Fat, g
ASDA			
Carrot & beetroot salad	160g (1 pack)	102	6.6
Cheese layered salad	440g (1 pack)	664	34
Mediterranean orzo pasta salad	280g (1 pack)	571	38
Prawn layered pasta salad	197g (1 pack)	276	14
Tuna layered pasta salad	440g (1 pack)	541	21
TESCO			
Caesar salad	230g (1 pack)	330	22
Chargrilled chicken pasta snack salad	275g (1 pack)	425	16
Cheese & tomato pasta snack salad	300g (1 pack)	545	21
Chicken & bacon layered salad	360g (1 pack)	600	40
Chilli chicken noodle salad	230g (1 pack)	165	2.5
Honey & mustard chicken pasta snack salad	350g (1 pack)	825	41
Prawn layered salad	380g (1 pack)	510	28
Spicy chilli chicken snack salad	350g (1 pack)	435	10
Tomato chicken pasta meal salad	260g (1 pack)	450	21
Tuna & sweetcorn snack salad	350g (1 pack)	680	28
FLORETTE			
Bistro salad	100g	27	0.2
Crispy salad	100g	22	0.3
Garden side salad	110g (1 pack)	26	0.3
Mixed salad	100g	20	0.2

*No information available
Tr trace quantities<0.1g

Saturated fat, g	Carbohydrate, g	Protein, g	Fibre, g
0.4	9.0	1.4	1.6
*	62	23	*
3.1	49	9.0	8.7
*	27	9.0	*
*	56	28	*
1.6	22	8.8	3.2
2.1	49	17	6.1
4.2	69	17	5.1
4.0	44	17	6.5
0.5	16	19	6.9
5.7	87	24	4.8
2.3	46	16	6.5
0.8	65	18	3.9
2.1	45	18	3.9
2.9	79	23	6.0
Tr	3.4	1.6	2.8
Tr	3.4	1.5	3.0
Tr	3.2	1.4	2.2
0.1	3.4	1.3	3.0

Sauces & dressings	Av Portion	Calories	Fat, g
Apple chutney	30g (1 tbsp)	57	0
Barbecue sauce	20g (1 tbsp)	19	0
Branston pickle, Crosse & Blackwell	30g (1 tbsp)	33	0.1
Brown sauce	20g (1 tbsp)	20	0
Chilli sauce	20g (1 tbsp)	16	0
French dressing	15g (1 tbsp)	98	11
Horseradish sauce	20g (1 tbsp)	31	2.0
Light mayonnaise, Hellman's	30g (1 tbsp)	88	8.9
Mango chutney	30g (1 tbsp)	57	0
Mayonnaise	30g (1 tbsp)	207	23
Salad cream	20g (1 tbsp)	70	6.0
Soy sauce	15g (1 tbsp)	10	0
Tomato ketchup	20g (1 tbsp)	23	0
PASTA SAUCE			
Bertolli pasta sauce with basil	100g	71	4.6
Dolmio bolognese	100g	50	1.3
Lloyd Grossman Tomato & chilli	100g	88	5.7
Seeds of Change Tomato & basil	100g	59	2.0
PESTO SAUCE			
Sacla classic green pesto	25g	138	11
Sacla sundried tomato pesto	25g	76	7.3
White sauce for lasagne, Dolmio	100g	98	7.5

*No information available
Tr trace quantities<0.1g

Saturated fat, g	Carbohydrate, g	Protein, g	Fibre, g
0	15	0.3	0.4
0	4.7	0.2	0.1
0	7.8	0.2	0.3
0	5.0	0.2	0.1
0	3.5	0.3	0.2
1.5	0	0	0
0.2	3.6	0.5	0.5
0.9	2.0	0.2	0
0	15	0.2	*
3.4	0.5	0.3	0
0.7	3.3	0.3	0
0	1.2	0.8	0
0	5.7	0.3	0.2
0.6	5.4	1.5	1.2
0.2	7.3	1.5	1.3
0.7	7.3	1.7	0.9
0.4	9.0	1.2	0.8
1.1	1.0	1.4	1.3
1.1	1.4	1.1	1.1
2.8	6.9	0.5	

Soft drinks	Av Portion	Calories	Fat, g
JUICE			
Apple juice	200ml	76	0
Cranberry juice	200ml	98	0
Grape juice	200ml	92	0
Grapefruit juice	200ml	66	0
Orange juice	200ml	72	0
Orange juice, freshly squeezed	200ml	66	0
Pineapple juice	200ml	82	0
Tomato juice	200ml	28	0
SQUASH & FRUIT DRINKS			
Barley water	250ml	35	0
Blackcurrant juice drink, made up	250ml	75	0
Capri Sun apple juice drink	200ml	92	0
Capri Sun orange juice drink	200ml	88	0
Elderflower cordial	250ml	67	0
Feel Good, orange & mango still juice drink	275ml bottle	110	0
Fruit Shoot, blackcurrant & apple	200ml	92	0
Fruit Shoot, low sugar, blackcurrant & apple	200ml	10	0
Fruit squash, made up	250ml	48	0
Glaceau Vitamin Water, all flavours	500ml bottle	95	0
High-juice drink, made up	250ml	63	0
Low calorie fruit squash, made up	250ml	3	0
Ribena	250ml	108	0

*No information available
Tr trace quantities<0.1g

Saturated fat, g	Carbohydrate, g	Protein, g	Fibre, g
0	20	0.2	0
0	23	0	0
0	23	0.6	0
0	17	0.8	0
0	19	1 0	0.2
0	16	1.2	0 2
0	21	0.6	0
0	6.0	1.6	1.2
0	9.3	0.3	0
0	20	0	0
0	22	0	0
0	21	0	0
0	17	0	0
0	25	0.5	0.5
0	22	0	0
0	1.6	0.2	0
0	13	0	0
0	23	0	0
0	17	0.3	0
0	0.5	0	0
0	26	0	0

Soft drinks	Av Portion	Calories	Fat, g
FIZZY DRINKS			
7 Up	330ml, 1 can	135	0
7 Up Free	330ml, 1 can	6	0
Appletiser sparkling apple juice	330ml bottle	162	0
Cola	330ml, 1 can	135	0
Diet cola	330ml, 1 can	3	0
Fanta orange	330ml, 1 can	99	0
Fruitiser, pomegranate & raspberry	330ml bottle	152	0
Ginger ale	150ml, 1 bottle	23	0
Irn Bru	330ml, 1 can	142	0
J2O, apple & mango	330ml bottle	142	0
J2O, orange & passion fruit	330ml bottle	155	0
Lemonade	330ml, 1 can	73	0
Orangina	330ml, 1 bottle	139	0
Orangina light	330ml, 1 bottle	20	0
Schloer sparkling red grape juice	250ml	105	0
Schloer sparkling white grape juice	250ml	105	0
Sprite	330ml, 1 can	145	0
Sprite zero	330ml, 1 can	3	0
Tango apple	330ml, 1 can	33	0
Tango orange	330ml, 1 can	63	0
Tonic water	150ml, 1 bottle	50	0
Vimto fizzy	330ml, 1 can	147	0

*No information available
Tr trace quantities<0.1g

Saturated fat, g	Carbohydrate, g	Protein, g	Fibre, g
0	35	0	0
0	0.3	0	0
0	39	0	0
0	36	0	0
0	0	0	0
0	23	0	0
0	38	0	0
0	5.9	0	0
0	35	0	0
0	33	0	0
0	36	0	0
0	19	0	0
0	33	0	0
0	4.0	0	0
0	26	0	0
0	26	0	0
0	35	0	0
0	0	0	0
0	7.0	0	0
0	14	0	0
0	13	0	0
0	36	0	0

Soft drinks	Av Portion	Calories	Fat, g
ENERGY DRINKS			
Lucozade energy, orange	380ml, 1 bottle	266	0
Monster energy drink	500ml, 1 can	228	0
Powerade energy, berry	500ml, 1 bottle	220	0
Red Bull	250ml, 1 can	113	0
Red Bull sugar-free	250ml, 1 can	8	0
Relentless	500ml, 1 can	230	0
SPORTS DRINKS			
Gatorade, orange	500ml, 1 bottle	120	0
Lucozade Sport Lite orange	500ml, 1 bottle	50	0
Lucozade Sport orange	500ml, 1 bottle	140	0
Powerade Zero berry & tropical fruit	500ml, 1 bottle	5	0
Powerade berry & tropical fruit	500ml, 1 bottle	80	0
Powerade cherry	500ml, 1 bottle	120	0

*No information available
Tr trace quantities<0.1g

Saturated fat, g	Carbohydrate, g	Protein, g	Fibre, g
0	65	0	0
0	57	0	0
0	53	0	0
0	28	0	0
0	3.0	0	0
0	52	0	0
0	30	0	0
0	10	0	0
0	32	0	0
0	0	0	0
0	20	0	0
0	29	0	0

Soft drinks	Av Portion	Calories	Fat, g
SMOOTHIES			
Innocent kiwi, apple & lime	250ml, 1 bottle	133	Tr
Innocent mango & passion fruit	250ml, 1 bottle	140	0.8
Innocent pineapple, banana & coconut	250ml, 1 bottle	193	3.5
Innocent strawberry & banana	250ml, 1 bottle	143	Tr
Innocent superfruit	250ml, 1 bottle	143	0.8
MILK DRINKS			
For Goodness Shakes chocolate	500ml, 1 bottle	316	5.4
For Goodness Shakes vanilla	500ml, 1 bottle	266	1.4
Frijj milkshake banana	500ml, 1 bottle	325	4.5
Frijj milkshake strawberry	500ml, 1 bottle	325	4.5
Slim Fast classic milkshake	325ml, 1 bottle	220	7.0
Slim Fast simply vanilla milkshake	325ml, 1 bottle	220	7.0
Yazoo milk drink banana	200ml, 1 bottle	130	2.4
Yazoo milk drink chocolate	200ml, 1 bottle	140	3.0
Yazoo milk drink strawberry	200ml, 1 bottle	130	2.4

*No information available
Tr trace quantities<0.1g

Saturated fat, g	Carbohydrate, g	Protein, g	Fibre, g
Tr	30	1.0	3.5
0.3	37	1.3	4.3
3.0	37	1.8	2.5
Tr	37	1.5	3.8
0.3	40	1.3	3.3
3.2	52	17	1.9
0.4	50	17	0.2
2.5	55	19	0
2.5	55	19	0
1.5	24	14	4.0
1.5	24	14	4.0
1.8	20	6.0	1.6
2.0	22	6.4	1.2
1.8	20	6.0	1.6

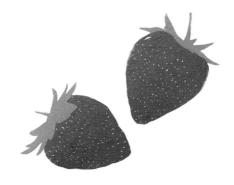

Soups	Av Portion	Calories	Fat, g
NEW COVENT GARDEN			
Broccoli & stilton	300g (½ carton)	167	11
Carrot & coriander	300g (½ carton)	129	6.6
Leek & potato	300g (½ carton)	150	6.0
Minestrone	300g (½ carton)	111	2.7
Spicy butternut squash & sweet potato	300g (½ carton)	192	11
Tomato & basil	300g (½ carton)	132	6.0
HEINZ			
Cream of chicken	200g (½ can)	105	6.0
Cream of mushroom	200g (½ can)	106	5.5
Cream of tomato	200g (½ can)	113	5.9
Vegetable	200g (½ can)	89	1.7
WEIGHT WATCHERS			
Carrot & lentil	295g (1 can)	86	0.4
Chicken	295g (1 can)	98	3.1
Tomato	295g (1 can)	74	1.4
BAXTERS			
Country garden	200g (½ can)	73	1.2
Lentil & vegetable	200g (½ can)	87	0.4
Oxtail	200g (½ can)	93	2.7
Scotch broth	200g (½ can)	96	2.0
BATCHELORS CUP A SOUP			
Chicken & vegetable	27.5g (1 sachet)	137	6.6
Minestrone	23.5g (1 sachet)	93	1.8
Mushroom	24g (1 sachet)	123	6.3
Tomato	23.3g (1 sachet)	90	2.1

*No information available
Tr trace quantities<0.1g

Saturated fat, g	Carbohydrate, g	Protein, g	Fibre, g
6.9	0.1	8.7	3.3
3.9	16	1.8	3.6
3.6	20	3.6	2.4
0.3	17	4.2	3.6
4.5	21	3.0	3.0
0.9	16	3.9	3.9
1.0	9.4	3.4	0.2
0.8	11	3.4	0.3
0.4	13	1.8	0.8
0.1	16	2.2	1.8
0.1	17	3.8	2.1
0.4	13	4.7	0.1
0.1	13	2.0	0.8
0.6	14	1.9	1.7
0.1	16	4.8	2.3
0.6	13	3.9	1.0
0.8	16	4.0	1.3
3.3	18	1.3	2.2
0.9	17	1.9	1.3
3.7	15	1.1	0.5
1.1	16	0.9	0.8

Spreads	Av Portion	Calories	Fat, g
SWEET SPREADS			
Cadbury's milk chocolate spread	15g (1 tbsp)	86	5.6
Nutella hazelnut and chocolate spread	15g (1 tbsp)	80	4.7
Fruit spread	15g (1 tbsp)	18	0
Honey	20g (1 tbsp)	58	0
Jam, fruit with seeds	15g (1 tbsp)	39	0
Jam, stone fruit	15g (1 tbsp)	39	0
Lemon curd	15g (1 tbsp)	42	1.0
Marmalade	15g (1 tbsp)	39	0
Reduced sugar jam, Weight Watcher's, apricot	15g (1 tbsp)	24	0
SAVOURY SPREADS			
Cheese spread	15g (1 tbsp)	40	3.0
Dairylea cheese spread	25g (1 tbsp)	59	4.9
Dairylea cheese triangles	17.5g (1 triangle)	43	3.3
Dairylea light cheese triangles	17.5g (1 triangle)	26	1.2
Fish paste	10g (2 tsp)	17	1.0
The Laughing Cow cheese portions	17.5g (1 portion)	42	3.3
Liver pâté	40g (1 tbsp)	139	13
Marmite	4g (1 tsp)	9	0
Meat spread	10g (2 tsp)	19	1.0
Peanut butter, smooth	20g (1 tbsp)	121	10
Peanut butter, wholegrain	20g (1 tbsp)	121	11
Yeast extract	4g (1 tsp)	7	0
Fish paste	10g (2 tsp)	17	1.0

*No information available
Tr trace quantities<0.1g

Saturated fat, g	Carbohydrate, g	Protein, g	Fibre, g
*	8.1	0.6	*
1.5	8.5	1.0	0.5
0	4.7	0.1	*
0	15	0.1	0
0	10	0.1	*
0	10	0.1	*
0.2	9.4	0.1	0
0	10	0	0
0	5.8	0	0.2
2.4	0.7	1.7	0
3.2	1.1	2.7	0
2.2	1.1	2.0	0
0.8	1.0	2.6	0
*	0.4	1.5	0
2.3	1.0	1.9	0
3.8	0.3	5.0	0
0	0.8	1.5	0.1
0.6	0.2	1.6	0
2.6	2.6	4.5	1.1
1.9	1.5	5.0	1.2
*	0.1	1.6	0
*	0.4	1.5	0

Storecupboard ingredients	Av Portion, g	Calories	Fat, g
FLOURS			
Cornflour	20g (1 tbsp)	71	0
Flour, white, bread	20g (1 tbsp)	68	0
Flour, white, plain	20g (1 tbsp)	68	0
Flour, white, self-raising	20g (1 tbsp)	66	0
Flour, wholemeal	20g (1 tbsp)	62	0
SUGARS			
Golden syrup	20g (1 tbsp)	60	0
Sugar, brown	5g (1 tsp)	18	0
Sugar, icing	15g (1 tbsp)	59	0
Sugar, white	5g (1 tsp)	20	0
HERBS & SPICES			
Balsamic vinegar	15g (1 tbsp)	10	0
Basil, dried	1g (1 tsp)	3	0
Curry powder	2g (1 tsp)	5	0
Mixed herbs	2g (1 tsp)	5	0
Mustard powder	3g (1 tsp)	14	1.0
Mustard, smooth	8g (1 tsp)	11	1.0
Mustard, wholegrain	8g (1 tsp)	11	1.0
Salt	5g (1 tsp)	0	0
Stock cubes, Oxo, beef	7g (1 cube)	19	0.4
Stock cubes, Oxo, vegetable	7g (1 cube)	18	0.3
Tomato purée	20g (1 tbsp)	15	0
Vegetable bouillon powder, Marigold	5g (1 tsp)	12	0.4
Vinegar	15 (1 tbsp)	3	0

*No information available
Tr trace quantities<0.1g

Saturated fat, g	Carbohydrate, g	Protein, g	Fibre, g
0	18	0.1	0
0	15	2.3	0.6
0	16	1.9	0.6
0	15	1.8	0.6
0	13	2.5	1.8
0	16	0.1	0
0	5.1	0	0
0	16	0	0
0	5.3	0	0
0	2.5	Tr	0
0	0.4	0.1	*
0	0.5	0.2	0.5
0	0.7	0.2	*
0	0.6	0.9	*
0	0.8	0.6	*
0	0.3	0.7	0.4
0	0	0	0
Tr	3.0	1.1	Tr
0.2	2.9	0.7	0.1
0	2.8	1.0	0.6
0.2	1.5	0.5	Tr
0	0.1	0.1	0

Takeaways	Av Portion	Calories	Fat, g
FISH AND CHIPS			
Chips, fried vegetable oil	165g	394	20
Cod in batter	180g	445	28
Haddock in batter	220g	510	31
Plaice in batter	200g	514	34
Rock salmon in batter	125g	369	27
INDIAN			
Chicken curry	400g	580	39
Chicken tikka masala	400g	628	42
Naan bread	160g	456	12
Pilau rice	250g	543	29
Poppadums	20g	100	8.0
Prawn curry	350g	410	30
Samosa, meat	70g	190	12
Samosa, vegetable	70g	152	7.0
Vegetable curry	200g	210	15
CHINESE			
Beef chow mein	350g	476	21
Chicken chow mein	350g	515	25
Chicken satay	200g	382	21
Crispy duck	200g	662	48
Fried noodles	230g	352	26
Plain noodles	230g	143	1.0
Prawn crackers	70g	399	27
Sweet & sour chicken	400g	776	40

*No information available
Tr trace quantities<0.1g

Saturated fat, g	Carbohydrate, g	Protein, g	Fibre, g
5.9	50	5.3	3.6
7.4	21	29	0.9
8.1	22	38	0.9
9.0	24	30	1.0
6.6	13	18	0.5
12	10	47	8.0
15	10	52	6.4
1.6	80	13	3.2
*	64	6.8	1.5
1.6	5.7	2.3	1.2
4.9	7.7	29	7.0
3.1	13	8.0	1.7
*	21	3.6	1.8
3.0	15	5.0	*
4.5	51	23	*
4.1	44	30	3.9
6.0	6.0	43	4.4
14	0.6	56	0
*	26	4.4	1.2
0.2	30	5.5	1.6
2.5	41	0.2	0.8
5.2	79	30	*

Vegetables	Av Portion	Calories	Fat, g
Asparagus	80g	20	0.6
Aubergine	80g	12	0.3
Beansprouts	80g	25	0.4
Beetroot	80g	29	0.1
Broccoli	80g	26	1.0
Broccoli, sprouting	80g	28	1.0
Brussels sprouts	80g	34	1.0
Cabbage	80g	21	1.0
Cabbage, red	80g	17	0.3
Carrots	80g	28	0.3
Cauliflower	80g	27	1.0
Celeriac	80g	14	0.3
Celery	30g (1 stick)	2	Tr
Courgette	80g	14	0.3
Cucumber	25g (6 slices)	3	Tr
Curly kale	80g	26	1.0
Fennel	80g	10	1.3
Garlic	3g (1 clove)	3	Tr
Ginger	5g	2	Tr
Green beans	80g	18	1.0
Leeks	80g	18	1.0
Lettuce	20g	3	Tr
Marrow	80g	10	Tr
Mushrooms	80g	10	1.0
Onions	120g (one)	43	Tr
Parsnips	80g	51	1.0

*No information available
Tr trace quantities<0.1g

Saturated fat, g	Carbohydrate, g	Protein, g	Fibre, g
0.1	1.6	2.3	1.4
0.1	1.8	0.7	1.6
0.1	3.2	2.3	1.2
Tr	6.1	1.4	1.5
0.2	1.4	3.5	2.1
0.2	2.1	3.1	2.8
0.2	3.3	2.8	3.3
0.1	3.3	1.4	1.9
Tr	3.0	0.9	2.0
0.1	6.3	0.5	1.9
0.2	2.4	2.9	1.4
*	1.8	1.0	3.0
0	0.3	0.2	0.3
0.1	1.4	1.4	0.7
0	0.4	0.2	0.2
0.2	1.1	2.7	2.5
0.2	1.4	0.7	1.9
0	0.5	0.2	0.1
0	0.5	0.1	*
0.1	2.3	1.4	1.9
0.1	2.3	1.3	1.8
0	0.3	0.2	0.2
0	1.8	0.4	0.4
0.1	0.3	1.4	0.9
0	9.5	1.4	1.7
0.1	10	1.4	3.7

Vegetables	Av Portion	Calories	Fat, g
Parsnips, roast	80g	91	5.0
Peas, frozen	80g	53	1.0
Peppers, green	160g (one)	24	1.0
Peppers, red	160g (one)	51	1.0
Peppers, yellow	160g (one)	42	Tr
Plantain	150g (one)	176	1.0
Potatoes, baked	180g (one)	94	0.4
Potatoes, boiled	180g	130	0.1
Potatoes, chips, home-made	165g	312	11
Potatoes, chips, frozen, fried	165g	450	22
Potatoes, mashed with margarine	120g	125	5.0
Potatoes, new	80g	60	1.0
Potatoes, roast	130g	194	6.0
Potatoes, oven chips, frozen, baked	165g	259	7.0
Pumpkin	80g	10	1.0
Radishes	8g (one)	1	Tr
Runner beans	80g	18	1.0
Spinach	80g	20	1.0
Spring greens	80g	26	1.0
Spring onions	10g (one)	2	Tr
Squash, butternut	80g	29	Tr
Swede	80g	19	Tr
Sweet potatoes	180g (one)	157	1.0
Sweetcorn, canned	80g	98	1.0
Tomatoes, canned	200g (½ can)	32	Tr
Tomatoes	85g (one)	14	1.0

*No information available
Tr trace quantities<0.1g

Saturated fat, g	Carbohydrate, g	Protein, g	Fibre, g
Tr	10	1.3	3.8
0.2	7.4	4.6	4.1
0.2	4.2	1.3	2.6
0.2	10	1.6	2.6
Tr	8.5	1.9	2.7
0.2	44	1.7	1.9
Tr	22	2.7	1.6
Tr	31	3.2	2.2
1.0	50	6.4	3.6
2.0	59	6.8	4.0
1.1	19	2.2	1.3
0.1	14	1.2	0.9
0.8	34	3.8	2.3
2.8	46	5.3	3.0
0.1	1.8	0.6	0.8
0	0.2	0.1	0.1
0.1	2.6	1.3	1.6
0.1	1.3	2.2	1.7
0.1	1.3	2.2	1.7
0	0.3	0.2	0.2
0	6.6	0.9	1.3
0	4.0	0.6	1.5
0.2	2.2	2.0	1.6
0.2	21	2.3	1.1
0	6.0	2.0	1.4
0.1	2.6	0.6	0.9

Vegetarian products	Av Portion	Calories	Fat, g
TOFU			
Cauldron organic tofu mince	100g	189	11
Cauldron original tofu	100g	85	4.2
Cauldron marinated tofu pieces	80g (½ pack)	182	14
QUORN			
Broccoli & cheese escalopes	120g (1 escalope)	251	14
Chicken-style pieces	75g (¼ pack)	86	2.0
Cottage pie	250g	167	2.5
Crispy nuggets	17g (1 nugget)	33	2.0
Family roast	91g (⅕ pack)	96	1.8
Fajita strips	70g (½ pack)	69	1.1
Fillets	52g (1 fillet)	55	0.8
Fishless fingers	28.5g (1 finger)	66	3.0
Mince	75g (¼ pack)	79	1.5
Mini sausage rolls	18g (1 roll)	48	2.2
Mozzarella & pesto escalope	120g (1 escalope)	260	16
Peppered steaks	98g (1 steak)	115	3.7
Pieces	87.5g (¼ pack)	100	2.3
Smoky bacon-style slices	37.5g (¼ pack)	82	6.1
Steak strips	75G (¼ pack)	81	1.8

*No information available
Tr trace quantities<0.1g

Saturated fat, g	Carbohydrate, g	Protein, g	Fibre, g
2.6	2.5	19	1.9
0.7	1.9	10	0.9
2.0	0.8	14	2.2
3.5	20	10	3.5
0.5	4.3	11	4.3
1.3	28	6.3	4.5
0.2	1.4	2.0	0.8
0.4	4.1	14	4.4
0.2	4.9	9.8	3.5
0.1	2.6	6.8	2.6
0.5	6.3	2.9	1.4
0.4	3.4	11	4.1
0.8	4.3	2.8	0.5
4.0	18	12	5.4
0.5	7.3	11	3.9
0.5	5.1	12	4.8
0.7	1.1	4.6	2.7
0.8	3.2	11	4.5

Vegetarian products	Av Portion	Calories	Fat, g
VEGETARIAN SAUSAGES			
Cauldron Lincolnshire sausages	50g (1 sausage)	79	4.4
Garden Gourmet vegetarian hot dogs	70g (2 sausages)	173	11
Linda McCartney Italian vegetarian sausages	100g (2 sausages)	152	5.6
Linda McCartney original sausages	50g (1 sausage)	101	4.4
Quorn Cumberland sausages	50g (1 sausage)	86	3.5
Quorn sausages	42g (1 sausage)	70	2.9
VEGETARIAN READY MEALS			
Cauldron Falafel	100g (½ pack)	305	19
Linda McCartney cannelloni	375g	386	12
Linda McCartney lasagne	360g	450	20
Linda McCartney sausage roll	57g (1 roll)	159	8.0
Linda McCartney vegetarian farmhouse pies	146g (1 pie)	379	23
Linda McCartney vegetarian roast	113g	227	12
Tesco meat-free cauliflower cheese grills	92.7g (1 grill)	220	12
Tesco meat-free nut cutlets	70g (1 cutlet)	240	16
Tesco meat-free vegetable fingers	49g (2 fingers)	110	4.9
VEGETARIAN BURGERS			
Cauldron mushroom burgers	87.5g (1 burger)	150	7.0
Linda McCartney cranberry & camembert burgers	88g (1 burger)	250	14
Linda McCartney mozzarella burger	90g (1 burger)	233	15
Linda McCartney vegetarian burgers	50g (1 burger)	62	1.5
Quorn burgers southern-style	63g (1 burger)	123	6.2
Quorn Sizzling burgers	80g (1 burger)	128	4.8
Tesco meat-free Mexican-style bean burgers	105g (1 burger)	225	9.2
Tesco meat-free vegetable quarterpounders	105g (1 burger)	210	8.9
Tesco Vegelicious bean burgers	75g (1 burger)	126	4.5

*No information available
Tr trace quantities<0.1g

Saturated fat, g	Carbohydrate, g	Protein, g	Fibre, g
0.3	2.0	7.8	1.3
1.3	4.9	13	1.1
3.1	6.9	17	3.4
1.8	4.1	11	0.8
0.3	6.0	6.8	1.8
0.3	4.9	5.3	1.5
1.6	23	7.5	6.0
6.4	50	13	3.7
10	45	23	5.2
3.1	15	7.5	0.9
11	34	8.5	2.4
0.9	7.6	21	0.7
3.2	22	5.2	2.2
2.1	16	5.6	2.7
0.5	13	1.8	1.8
0.4	14	7.0	1.3
1.4	11	19	4.7
2.2	8.7	19	3.7
0.5	5.4	7.9	2.9
0.8	9.1	6.7	1.9
2.4	5.6	14	2.4
0.5	25	6.0	7.6
0.9	27	3.6	3.3
0.5	7.0	14	1.5

Yoghurt	Av Portion	Calories	Fat, g
Alpro soya yoghurt, plain	100g (1 pot)	46	2.3
Danone Actimel drink, strawberry	100g (1 bottle)	75	1.5
Danone Activia 0%, raspberry	125g (1 pot)	59	0.1
Danone Activia creamy, strawberry	120g (1 pot)	117	3.6
Danone Activia pouring yoghurt, vanilla	130g	81	2.1
Danone Activia, strawberry	125g (1 pot)	116	4.0
Fat-free yoghurt, fruit	125g (1 pot)	59	0
Fat-free yoghurt, plain	125g (1 pot)	68	0
Greek-style yoghurt, fruit	125g (1 pot)	171	10
Greek-style yoghurt, plain	125g (1 pot)	166	13
Low-fat yoghurt, fruit	125g (1 pot)	98	1.0
Low-fat yoghurt, plain	125g (1 pot)	70	1.0
Müller Corner greek yoghurt, black cherry	150g (1 pot)	173	4.5
Müller Light, strawberry	175g (1 pot)	89	0.2
Müller Vitality yoghurt drink, raspberry	100g (1 bottle)	74	1.7
Whole milk yoghurt, fruit	150g (1 pot)	164	5.0
Whole milk, yoghurt, plain	150g (1 pot)	119	5.0
Yakult fermented milk drink	65g (1 bottle)	43	0
Yeo Valley organic yoghurt pots, strawberry	120g (1 pot)	123	4.4

Cream			
Clotted	30g (1 tbsp)	176	19
Crème fraiche	30g (1 tbsp)	113	12
Crème fraiche, half-fat	30g (1 tbsp)	49	5.0
Double	30g (1 tbsp)	149	16
Single	30g (1 tbsp)	58	6.0
Whipping	30g (1 tbsp)	114	12

*No information available
Tr trace quantities<0.1g

Saturated fat, g	Carbohydrate, g	Protein, g	Fibre, g
0.4	2.1	4.0	1.0
1.1	12	2.7	0
0	8.6	5.8	3.1
2.3	15	5.8	0.2
1.3	11	5.1	0
2.5	16	4.4	2.5
0	8.8	6.0	0
0	10	6.8	0
7.0	14	6.0	0
8.4	6.0	7.1	0
1.0	17	5.2	0.3
0.8	9.3	6.0	0
2.7	24	7.5	0.2
0.2	14	6.8	0.4
1.0	11	2.8	1.0
3.0	27	6.0	0
2.6	12	8.5	0
0	9.6	0.9	0
2.8	15	5.8	0.1
12	0.7	0.5	0
0.1	0.7	0.7	0
3.0	1.3	0.8	0
10	0.5	0.5	0
3.6	0.7	1.0	0
7.6	0.8	0.6	0

My calorie counting chart

MONDAY	WHAT I ATE TODAY	PORTION SIZE	CALORIES
Breakfast	Muesli with semi-skimmed milk	50g	210
	1 glass orange juice	200ml	72
Morning Snack	1 apple	100g	47
	Cappuccino	Tall	91
Lunch	Chicken salad sandwich		272
	1 banana	100g	95
	1 diet cola	330ml	3
Afternoon Snack	Carrot cake	75g	269
	3 dried apricots	40g	63
Dinner	Vegetable lasagne	400g	453
	Garden salad	110g	26
	1 low-fat fruit yoghurt	125g	98
	1 glass red wine	175ml	119
TOTAL CALORIES			1,818
CALORIES ALLOWED			2,000

TUESDAY	WHAT I ATE TODAY	PORTION SIZE	CALORIES
Breakfast	PORRIDGE	APPROX 30G	150
	WHITE TEA/SWEETNER		20
Morning Snack			
Lunch			
Afternoon Snack			
Dinner			
TOTAL CALORIES			
CALORIES ALLOWED			15

WEDNESDAY	WHAT I ATE TODAY	PORTION SIZE	CALORIES
Breakfast			
Morning Snack			
Lunch			
Afternoon Snack			
Dinner			
TOTAL CALORIES			
CALORIES ALLOWED			

THURSDAY	WHAT I ATE TODAY	PORTION SIZE	CALORIES
Breakfast			
Morning Snack			
Lunch			
Afternoon Snack			
Dinner			
TOTAL CALORIES			
CALORIES ALLOWED			

FRIDAY	WHAT I ATE TODAY	PORTION SIZE	CALORIES
Breakfast			
Morning Snack			
Lunch			
Afternoon Snack			
Dinner			
TOTAL CALORIES			
CALORIES ALLOWED			

Body Mass Index (BMI chart)

Use this chart to find out your Body Mass Index (BMI). First find your height (in feet and inches) on the left hand side of the chart. Then follow the row along until you reach your weight (in stones and pounds). Select the nearest value/s to your own if they are not displayed in the chart. Your BMI will be listed at the top of the chart.

BMI	19	20	21	22	23	24	25	26	27	28	29	30	31	32	33	34	35
Height (ins)	**Body Weight (stone)**																
4 10"	6.5	6.9	7.1	7.5	7.9	8.2	8.5	8.9	9.2	9.6	9.9	10.2	10.6	10.9	11.3	11.6	12.0
4 11"	6.7	7.1	7.4	7.8	8.1	8.5	8.9	9.1	9.5	9.9	10.2	10.6	10.9	11.2	11.6	12.0	12.3
5	6.9	7.3	107	7.6	8.4	8.8	9.1	9.5	9.9	10.2	10.6	10.9	11.3	11.6	12.0	12.4	12.8
5 1"	7.1	7.6	7.9	8.3	8.7	9.1	9.4	9.8	10.2	10.6	10.9	11.3	11.7	12.1	12.4	12.9	13.2
5 2"	7.4	7.8	8.2	8.6	9.0	9.4	9.7	10.1	10.5	10.9	11.3	11.7	12.1	12.5	12.9	13.3	13.6
5 3"	7.6	8.1	8.4	8.9	9.3	9.6	10.1	10.4	10.9	11.3	11.6	12.1	12.5	12.9	13.3	13.6	14.1
5 4"	7.9	8.3	8.7	9.1	9.6	10.0	10.4	10.8	11.2	11.6	12.1	12.4	12.9	13.3	13.7	14.1	14.6
5 5"	8.1	8.6	9.0	9.4	9.9	10.3	10.7	11.1	11.6	12.0	12.4	12.9	13.3	13.7	14.1	14.6	15.0
5 6"	8.4	8.9	9.3	9.7	10.1	10.6	11.1	11.5	11.9	12.4	12.8	13.3	13.7	14.1	14.6	15	15.4
5 7"	8.6	9.1	9.6	10.0	10.4	10.9	11.4	11.9	12.3	12.7	13.2	13.6	14.1	14.6	15.1	15.5	15.9
5 8"	8.9	9.4	9.9	10.3	10.8	11.3	11.7	12.2	12.6	13.1	13.6	14.1	14.5	15.0	15.4	15.9	16.4
5 9"	9.1	9.6	10.1	10.6	11.1	11.6	12.1	12.6	13.0	13.5	14.0	14.5	14.9	15.4	15.9	16.4	16.9
5 10"	9.4	9.9	10.4	10.9	11.4	11.9	12.4	12.9	13.4	13.9	14.4	14.9	15.9	16.4	16.9	17.4	
5 11"	9.7	10.2	10.7	11.2	11.8	12.3	12.8	13.3	13.8	14.3	14.9	15.4	15.9	16.4	16.9	17.4	17.9
6	10.0	10.5	11.0	11.6	12.1	12.6	13.1	13.6	14.2	14.7	15.2	15.8	16.3	16.8	17.3	17.9	18.4
6 1"	10.3	10.8	11.4	11.9	12.4	13.0	13.5	14.1	14.6	15.1	15.6	16.2	16.8	17.3	17.9	18.4	18.9
6 2"	10.6	11.1	11.4	12.2	12.8	13.3	13.9	14.4	15.0	15.6	16.1	16.6	17.2	17.8	18.3	18.9	19.4
6 3"	10.9	11.4	12.0	12.6	13.1	13.7	14.3	14.9	15.4	16.0	16.6	17.1	17.7	18.3	18.9	19.4	19.9
6 4"	11.1	11.7	12.3	12.9	13.5	14.1	14.6	15.2	15.8	16.4	17.0	17.6	18.1	18.8	19.4	19.9	20.5

Calorie swaps

By making a few easy swaps in your diet you can save calories and drop pounds. As a general rule, cut down on saturated fat (found in fatty meat, burgers, sausages, bacon, butter, pastry and puddings) and sugar (found in soft drinks, biscuits, cakes, confectionery and puddings). These foods are loaded with calories and are easy to over-consume without filing you up.

Instead, choose high fibre and low-medium fat foods that are rich in nutrients and naturally filling: fruit, vegetables, salad, lower fat dairy products, wholegrain cereals. Keep a check on portion sizes, especially when eating out, and always include the calories in drinks in your daily tally.

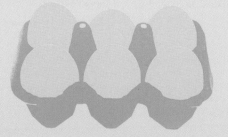

Swap	For this	Save
2 fried eggs	2 poached eggs	66 calories
1 slice cheesecake	1 pot low-fat fruit yogurt	122 calories
1 slice apple pie	Stewed apples with sugar (110g)	201 calories
1 bag crisps (30g)	30g plain popcorn	100 calories
1 flapjack	1 teacake	200 calories
2 crackers with 40g cheese	1 slice wholemeal toast with 1 tablespoon low-fat cheese	107 calories
1 rasher streaky bacon	1 rasher trimmed back bacon	40 calories
1 croissant	30g Bran Flakes with semi-skimmed milk	67 calories
1 Mars bar	1 banana	180 calories
50g raisins	50g grapes	106 calories
Cappuccino	'Skinny' cappuccino	46 calories
Chicken korma (350g)	Chicken tikka (350g)	230 calories

Useful websites

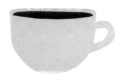

British Nutrition Foundation
www.nutrition.org.uk
The website of the British Nutrition Foundation contains information, fact sheets and educational resources on nutrition and health.

NHS Choices
www.nhs.uk/Livewell/healthy-eating
The NHS website has information on healthy eating, weight loss, food safety, food labelling, and health issues.

British Dietetic Association
www.bda.uk.com
The website of the British Dietetic Association includes fact sheets and information on healthy eating. It also provides details of Registered Dietitians working in private practice.

British Nutrition Foundation
www.nutrition.org.uk
The website of the British Nutrition Foundation provides food fact sheets for the general public on a wide range of nutrition and health topics.

Vegetarian Society
www.vegsoc.org
This website provides information on vegetarian nutrition and lifestyles as well as general nutrition, health and recipes.

Weight Concern
www.weightconcern.com
Weight Concern is a registered charity and their website provides excellent information on weight loss including a self-help Shape-Up programme

Beat (Beating Eating Disorders)
http://www.b-eat.co.uk
The website of Beat (the working name of the Eating Disorders Association) provides helplines, online support and a network of UK-wide self-help groups for adults and young people as well as information sheets and booklets, which can be downloaded free.

Health Supplements Information Service www.hsis.org
This website provides information on vitamins, minerals and health supplements.

The Mayo Clinic
www.mayoclinic.com
Written by medical experts, this US site offers good nutrition and health information, as well as advice on medical conditions in a user-friendly format.

Ediets
www.ediets.com
This website provides personalised diet plans, as well as health and fitness features, recipes and on-line support

Weight Loss Resources
www.weightlossresources.co.uk
This UK website provides excellent information on weight loss, fitness and healthy eating as well as a comprehensive calorie database and a personalised weight loss programme.

WebMD
www.webmd.com
This comprehensive US website has an A – Z directory of health topics and advice on many aspects of nutrition and fitness.

The British Heart Foundation
www.bhf.org.uk
This website contains user-friendly information on keeping your heart healthy, healthy eating, exercise, fitness and preventing heart disease.

Diabetes UK
www.diabetes.org.uk
Diabetes UK is the leading charity for people with diabetes and this website provides authoritative information on diabetes, as well as a support network and sections for children, teenagers and young adults

Health Status
www.healthstatus.com
This US website provides useful health calculators and assessments that help you work out your body mass index, body fat percentage, number of calories burned during exercise and daily calorie intake.

Nutrition Data
http://nutritiondata.self.com/
This US website provides a detailed nutrition database together with nutritional information from food manufacturers and restauarants.

Net Doctor
www.netdoctor.co.uk/dietandnutrition
This UK website provides excellent advice on healthy eating, weight loss, health conditions, weight problems and lifestyle management

First published in the United Kingdom in 2013 by
Collins & Brown
10 Southcombe Street
London
W14 0RA

An imprint of Anova Books Company Ltd

Nutritional date sourced from
UK Nutrient Databank

Illustrations by Marcus Butt

The Good Housekeeping website is www.allboutyou.com/goodhousekeeping

10 9 8 7 6 5 4 3 2

ISBN 978-1-908449-26-9

A catalogue record for this book is available from the British Library.

Reproduction by Dot Gradations Ltd, UK
Printed and bound by G. Canale & C SpA, Italy

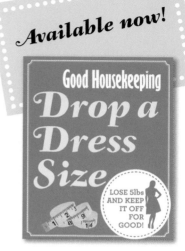

Available now!

Good Housekeeping
Drop a Dress Size

LOSE 5lbs
AND KEEP
IT OFF
FOR
GOOD!

This book can be ordered direct from the publisher at www.anovabooks.com

£10.99 | ISBN 978-1-908449-15-3